CW00549159

THE POWER IN SOFTNESS

THE POWER IN SOFTNESS

A Guide to Personal Protection and Empowerment
for Women

Charly Flower

THE POWER IN SOFTNESS

First Published 2011
Copyright© Charly Flower 2011
All Rights Reserved

ISBN 978-0-9567014-6-6

No part of this book may be reproduced in any form,
by photocopying or by any electronic or mechanical means,
including information storage or retrieval systems,
without permission in writing from the copyright
owner and the publisher of this book.

Printed In Great Britain by
Direct POD

I dedicate this book to Thea.
She is the softest and most powerful person
I have ever known.

CONTENTS

ABOUT THIS BOOK

This book is a collection of insights and reflections about the power in softness that came to me while working as a female bouncer. Each chapter comprises knowledge, exercises, and a corresponding story, or two, that I hope the reader will find interesting. These stories illustrate how I came to experience the truth of softness, in practice.

Some of these stories are allegorical, some might disturb, and some might raise a chuckle, but all of them illustrate an aspect of personal protection and empowerment that is relevant either physically, mentally, or spiritually. Some of the stories you might think are too physical to illustrate softness, but whether obvious or hidden, softness lies at the heart of each one – it is up to you to find it.

You will notice throughout that the attacker is referred to as "he". The reason for this is that this is a book for women. While I understand that women can be violent, the overwhelming majority of women are attacked by men. Domestic violence is more prevalent than ever: in the home, women are increasingly attacked by the men they live with. On the street, women are also attacked by men. I, personally, have never heard of a woman single-handedly stalking, or attacking another woman on the street. If it does happen at all, it is very rare.

The Power in Softness – A Guide to Personal Protection and Empowerment for Women, can be applied on three different levels: the physical, mental, and spiritual. If I have been able to reach women on any of these levels, I will have considered my job well done. To have touched them on all three would be a gift.

Once a woman is able to honour her physical, mental, and spiritual selves, she becomes more than the sum of these different parts: she becomes a true female warrior, and a powerful presence in the world.

This book represents a journey from hardness to softness. Its pages contain the entire spectrum of human emotion. Travelling from the hardness of masculine energy to the softness of the feminine, cannot properly be done without opening up our capacity to feel – in every sense. This particular journey has changed the map I use to guide me through life. The map I now use is unrecognisable from the first one.

May you walk in softness, and in safety.

C.F.

INTRODUCTION

I became a bouncer to prove to the world that I was powerful, that I could cut it with the best of them, and that I was tough. I decided one day that fifteen years of martial arts training, three black belts to my name, and a bodybuilding frame that could push over two hundred kilogrammes on the leg press, was all the qualification I needed to become a door supervisor. As I walked through the doors of my first club, I recall feeling that I had "arrived". Strutting around with my Security Industry Authority badge on, I would command respect and attention. The macho way of doing things was the way to go: to succeed, you had to be hard. My SIA badge gave me licence to carry on living this illusion.

In the film, *The Matrix*, Morpheus illuminates the truth about life to Neo. He explains that living the life for which we are programmed is to live an illusion. Being stuck in the illusion is a bit like being a fly caught in a spider's web: you are a prisoner. To be free means you must literally die to the version of yourself that you hold: your personality and identity are nothing more than a programme. As a bouncer, I was living in the matrix.

Then one day, the bubble burst. The illusion I had been trying so hard to uphold came crashing down around me. I discovered something so powerful and vast, that I couldn't understand how I hadn't been able to see it before. It had been right in front of me all along: it was the power in softness. How ironic to have hit upon the power in softness in the hardest of environments. Out of the darkness of a nightclub, a light emerged; a crack appeared in my perception that opened me to the notion that not everything had to be sorted out using force. No sooner had softness arrived, than things started to change and the matrix no longer had me.

It took courage to risk being vulnerable in what were sometimes dangerous situations on the doors. There were a few defining moments that will always stay with me, and they were instrumental in teaching me that softness really can melt anger and hate. The ease with which I was able to diffuse violence using the softly-softly approach, grew and grew. Before long, I was using softness in almost all of the dangerous confrontations I was involved in. Soon after that, I was a convert: I became softness itself. Softness is powerful stuff. I always liken it to the gentle action of washing-up liquid applied to grease. I never imagined that using it would be of any use against physical force – the Fairy Liquid take on violence proved me wrong.

As if this were not enough, the power in softness had yet another surprise – this one even more miraculous than the first. Soon after I had started working as a bouncer, I was diagnosed with an enormous benign tumour in my womb. I panicked for about two days, and then did something I had never done before: I went inside myself to a soft place and listened. I didn't try to solve the problem from the outside. At first, I heard a faint voice that grew louder as time went on. This voice took on the role of advisor, and as I began to trust it, its presence became a real force in my life. It advised me to surrender to my intuitions, dreams, and visions, and to let them direct me – this would be my path to healing. It also whispered that early on in my childhood, I had traded in softness and my sacred femininity for hardness and the masculine way of things. It spoke softly to me of how I needed to become whole and complete, and that I couldn't achieve this if I refused to acknowledge the softness within. The voice spoke of power, the true meaning of it, and the way to reclaim it. I yielded to this guidance, and I healed. I softened, then softened some more, and the tumour in my womb disappeared as quickly as it had arrived. For the first time, I understood the meaning of balance.

Central to my journey was a sense of power loss. Early on, I had experienced an alienation from my feminine roots and heritage. Later on, I made it my mission to get back that lost power. Once softness had arrived, it became obvious that I would never find that lost power in the world of hardness. This journey isn't unique: I have no doubt that many women have experienced power loss in this way. The truth is, as women, we can only get our power back by taking responsibility for what we really are, and by honouring our gifts of womanhood – anything less is a giveaway. We give our power away every time we collude with the world's obsession with form. Every time we agonize over our physical appearance, we lose a bit of our truth. Every time we allow the outer world to define us – at the expense of our inner knowing – we kill off a little bit more of our sacred femininity. Taking back our power is about having the courage to explore and hold not only our feelings, perceptions, intuitions, but our connection to the divine also. It is a matter of accepting our softness – that is where our power lies.

The power in softness and the way of the feminine are inextricably linked: the way of the feminine is the way of *being* and *experiencing,* but softness is the way to get there. Let us weave the thread of softness through everything: through our relationships, our work, and our inner being. As women, we are consummate weavers.

The modern world hasn't been ready for the emergence of the feminine, but it is now. I wondered long and hard about why when I was working on the doors, there was so much resistance to my being there. At first, I thought it was because I wasn't powerful enough. As time went on, I realized that it was because I was too powerful. Often, male colleagues would try and pretend I was invisible – not because I couldn't get the job done, but because I could. I had found out a secret: women have been silenced, not for their lack of power, but because of it.

I feel it is time for women to stop hiding. It is time for us to bring softness back into the world, and return balance to our sacred Mother Earth. It is time for us to be heard, as well as seen. And it is time for us to open to a power so much greater than any power already here. The power in softness can keep you safe. It can bring serenity and light into your world. It can help you navigate your way through each day effortlessly. It can even make a benign tumour the size of a melon disappear. I call that magic.

PROLOGUE

Women everywhere are more educated and informed than ever, about how we, the holders and keepers of knowledge, have become as strangers to our once cherished sacred feminine. Education and information alone, however, cannot resurrect our divine feminine heritage any more than merely talking about an illness can heal it.

Women of earth, let us move away from the masculinity of our minds, and rest within the femininity of our hearts. Let us become the softness there, and rewrite the book of earth to birth the "her-story" that has been bound, and gagged, for so long.

THE POWER IN
SOFTNESS

Chapter One

DANGERS IN CLUB LAND – SOME TIPS

MOBILE PHONES

Each time you give in to your mobile phone, you give your power away. If you don't have it in you to just let it ring whenever it goes off, then you are a slave to it, and your mobile phone has you. Remember, that as you walk in a public place, your greatest defence is awareness. If you are talking or texting on your mobile when you are out and about, you are much more likely to be attacked because your ability to notice has gone. As you chatter away, someone could so easily come up behind you and grab you. And bearing in mind that an average street attack lasts for about three seconds, what makes you think that under those circumstances you would have enough time to dial a number, wait for it to ring, and then scream for help? To make it home, leave your mobile phone alone.

A street mugger will only take something of yours he can see. He isn't going to steal from you unless he is absolutely sure you have the thing he wants. He doesn't have time to bet on the odds of you having a mobile phone. Years ago, I was out one evening when a young woman, who was only a few feet in front of me on the pavement, suddenly shrieked. A mugger had whizzed by on his bike and pinched the fancy new mobile phone that she had been speaking on only moments earlier. Before she could do anything about it, the mugger had sped off to another part of town. What struck me most about the incident was not that it had happened, but the fact that the young woman was so astounded that it had. Being jumped for your mobile phone is such an easy attack to prevent. Just slip the thing where the street thief can't see it: into your pocket or bag. "Out of sight, out of mind" is a tried, and tested, maxim for the street.

It isn't only your observational skills that must be keen on the street: you also need both hands free, should you need to defend yourself. If you are attacked on the street while talking on your mobile phone, how would you rate your chances of being able to do this with only one hand? I would say your odds are pretty slim.

While patrolling a busy dance floor one night, I was called to a fire escape: a young man lay unconscious on the stairs. Two men from a rival group had seized him from behind on the dance floor, and dragged him there to carry out one of the most ferocious attacks I'd ever seen on the doors. The lad had a deep gash to his forehead, and an ear so badly cut that it was hanging off. That was the least of my problems: the young man was losing so much blood that I feared for his life.

I wondered how he'd come to this. Soon after, I found out: he'd been standing facing a dark corner of the dance floor, talking on his mobile phone when the two thugs attacked. Taking advantage of the fact that the young lad couldn't see them coming, they grabbed him from behind and shoved him through an exit door at knife point.

The tragic events of the night hung around in my mind like a stale, rank miasma. On my way home, I visualized the attack again and again in the hope of being able to come to terms with the savagery of it – I so wanted to be able to turn the clock back. If only the young man had been facing the crowd instead of the dark corner, he might have seen his attackers coming.

I'd given up what ifs long ago, and anyway, I was home. Shaken and exhausted from the night's events, I opened my gate and walked up to my front door. Just as I was about to let myself in, my mobile rang. With my back to the street and facing the front door, I thought better of answering the call. I left it. I'd seen only too well what mobile phones can do. I'd seen how they demand all of your attention and make the world around you disappear. I, for one, had no intention of disappearing anywhere.

SUBSTANCE ABUSE

During my time on the doors, I began to notice that women were getting legless much more quickly than men. Science does back this up: exhaustive research has proven that equal amounts of alcohol will affect women far more rapidly than men. The speed at which it hits the female bloodstream goes off the chart compared to that of men. If you are on your way out to one of your favourite watering holes, have a care as to how much, and how fast, you consume alcohol. Being carried out over a bouncer's shoulder is often a very undignified affair – particularly if you have a short skirt on.

Substance abuse is simply inner abuse externalised.

"Charly! Get your arse down 'ere! There's a woman collapsed on the dance floor!" bellowed a pug-faced bar manager from the bottom of the stairs. It was the height of summer, and the heat downstairs inside the undersized nightclub was intolerable. "Throw 'er out or we'll 'ave the Battle of bloody Pearl 'Arbour down 'ere!" he yelled again, opening his mouth so wide that I could see his back molars.

The tiny club was now so over capacity, that the thought of having to squeeze my way through a fog of bodies dripping with sweat didn't inspire me. But, I reminded myself, these moments were a bouncer's lot. I gritted my teeth, raced downstairs, and disappeared into the crowd to find her.

And there she was: a woman in her early twenties, rolling about half naked right in the middle of the dance floor, with her miniskirt up to her armpits. She'd drunk herself senseless, fallen backwards, and was now only a step away from getting trampled on. I could see that helping the young woman to her feet would probably be a waste of time, but in the interests of saving myself the arduous ascent to the top of the stairs, with her over my shoulder, I had a go. As soon as I pulled her up, her legs went to jelly and she began a slow, elegant slide to the floor – as I'd predicted. She wasn't the only one to take a nosedive: gravity that night had got the better of quite a few party bashers – people were dropping like ninepins.

I quickly squatted low enough for the wobbly young woman to do a graceful flop over my shoulder, then straightened up. Holding her legs tight, I put out my hand to feel my way through the half-lit mass of steaming bodies to the staircase, and slowly began the upward climb. Using one hand to pull us both up with, and the other to keep the young woman's legs from flying apart, I took each step at a time, occasionally stopping to rest. As soon as I reached the top, I took her outside and carefully laid her down on the pavement by the front door. My escape from, what my colleagues and I often referred to as the Black Hole of Calcutta, was short lived. The bar manager wasn't done yet, and before I'd even had a chance to cool down, he was back at the bottom of the stairs exercising his larynx. "Charly! Come and get 'er blinkin' 'andbag! It's down 'ere on the bar!"

I flew back down into the blackness to get it. The bar manager handed me the bag with a scowl. "Make sure she don't bloody come back in! She's a f—g nightmare, that one!" he said, punching the air with an uncorked bottle of wine and spilling it all over the bar.

I tucked the young woman's handbag under my arm and ran back upstairs. And there she was, retching in the gutter. A friend of hers approached and gasped at the sight of her closest chum, face down in cigarette butts and dog turd, throwing up all over the pavement. I took the friend to one side. "Tomorrow," I said, "I want you to tell your girlfriend every single detail about what she did tonight. Tell her how she ended up in the gutter. Be graphic – don't leave out a thing." Until you become conscious of a self-destructive pattern, you can't fix it.

FOOTWEAR

If I had been given a penny for all the times I have told women to put their shoes back on while on the dance floor, I would be rolling in it. So many women wear high heels when they go out clubbing, and so many of them take them off at some point in the evening. If you are so uncomfortable wearing them that you have to walk around barefoot, then take a pair of trainers with you to a club and change into them as soon as you get there. Granted, rubber soles might not be the height of fashion, but they are the more practical choice. Even the most civilized of club floors is littered with broken glass. Trainers are also the safer choice for the street – particularly when you are walking home alone late at night. Rubber soles make less noise than high heels do, so you can't be heard coming. They are also so quiet that you can hear someone's footsteps behind you, should you be followed. And of course with trainers on, you can always leg it at full speed – should you need to.

While checking the ladies' toilet one night, I noticed a woman sitting on a

*stool swinging her high heels from her fingers, and looking thoroughly
cheesed off. I asked her why she wasn't out on the dance floor having fun.
"My feet are killin' me," she moaned. "They're swollen and I need to rest
'em. I wish I 'adn't worn these," she sighed, twirling one of her pearl
encrusted stilettos in the air for me to admire. "I can't resist wearing 'em,
though, as they're so flatterin'," she continued, trying to squeeze her puffy
feet back into them. "It's stupid, innit? I can't even run in 'em if some
geezer is after me!"*

*All high heels should come with a government health warning: "These
shoes are hazardous to your health and could seriously endanger your
safety."*

THE DANGER OF MIXED MESSAGES

A man doesn't interpret verbal cues in the same way that a woman does. In a
man's world, yes means yes, and no is a definite *no*. Notice what happens next
time a man asks you something. If your answer is no, are you smiling as you
say it? To a man, a no with a smile is actually a yes. At the very least, smiling
when saying no will imply that you aren't sure, or that your no could well be a
perhaps. In future, have a go at not smiling each time you say no – see where
that leads. A man rarely smiles when saying it, so why not apply the same rules
that he does?

People are far more influenced by what they see, than by what they hear. If a
stranger asks you for a dance, he won't be taking his cue from your answer –
from what you say. He will be taking it from how you respond bodily – from
what you do. If you answer with a "no thank you" and deliver a radiant smile as
you say it, the stranger will probably still move in because to him, your smile is
the green light he is waiting for. If you want a stranger to take your no for an
answer, don't cancel it out with a smile. Keep all your woman-to-man one-
liners crystal clear, and never give a man two messages where one will do.

Two very beautiful women walked in through the doors one night: men

everywhere turned to stare at them as they gracefully sauntered by. Some of this attention was unwelcome for one of the beauties; she struggled with it all, while her friend didn't. After shadowing them for a bit it was easy to see why: when asked to dance, the beauty having all the problems would go overboard so as not to offend. Each time she refused a dance, she'd smile sweetly, flick her hair this way and that, and end things with a "perhaps", or a "maybe". This is no help to an alpha male on the prowl: the men pursuing her understood this to be open season, and would be back.

After a few hours of unrelenting badgering from predatory males, the young beauty had finally had enough. One man in particular had been following her for most of the evening and was beginning to unsettle her – it was time to get help. I was stationed upstairs keeping an eye on the dance floor below, when I spotted the young beauty looking up at me. She recognized me as a member of security, waved to get my attention, and daintily hurried up the stairs to ask me what to do. "If you want him to go away," I recommended, "don't feel as if you need to spare his feelings." All of the young woman's froth and sparkle immediately went flat – I could have been suggesting that she drown a kitten. To her, being totally honest with someone was tantamount to being openly aggressive. I had a go at explaining the difference. "You can tell someone how you feel without being harsh," I said, gently. The fragile-looking woman didn't seem convinced. "Do you want to spend time with him?" I asked. The young beauty lowered her eyes and, as if ashamed of herself for saying it, mumbled a quiet no. "Then why don't you tell him that?" I said.

I hadn't expected her to take my advice quite so literally. She took a deep breath and walked straight up to the man who'd been stalking her for most of the night. She tapped him delicately on the shoulder, looked him in the eye, and delivered a completely uncensored version of what she truly felt. "Please don't bother me again. I don't want to be with you because I do not find you attractive." The man went as white as a sheet: both softness and directness coexisting in one person was more than he could handle. Clubbers had now stopped to delight in an unexpected bit of entertainment – the man was fast becoming a laughing stock. Unfortunately for him, there was more. With a firm, but mild-mannered tone, the beautiful young woman finished what she'd started. "You are not my type. Pardon me for mentioning it, but you do look as if you need a bath. If you ever come near me again, I will repeat all this much, much louder."

No smiles, no frills, no added extras, and no more men on her tail.

SPIKING

Spiking is a way of life these days: if four women go out drinking to a bar or a club, the odds are that one of them will have her drink spiked. The only way to be certain that your drink hasn't been tampered with is to make sure that you never take your eyes off it – what's yours is yours and no one else's. If you need to move away from where you are, then take your glass with you. And one more thing: never accept a cigarette from a stranger. Men have taken to spiking those as well.

It is a terrible thing to wake up in a stranger's bed and not know how you got there, or what happened. Rohypnol is nasty stuff: it interrupts the body's ability to coordinate. Just the tiniest amount of it will send you gaga and floppy, and you will have absolutely no defence against a stranger who is about to walk you out of a bar, then drive you home – to his place.

On a routine patrol of the ladies' room one night, I found a young woman being sick in a toilet. With one shoe missing, and a face smeared with running mascara and lipstick, she flopped back against the cubicle wall and lay, hunched over, in a pool of her own vomit. Worried that she might be losing consciousness, I bent down to help her to her feet and as I did, she grabbed my tie, pulled me close, and whispered, "Drink, sp—" The young woman seemed desperate to share something, but whatever it was would have to wait: the atmosphere in the ladies' room was stifling – it was time to get her outside for a bit of cold night air.

With one hand around the young woman's waist, and my shoulder tucked snugly under her armpit, I walked her all the way to the entrance. Before taking her out, I propped her up against the wall just inside the front door, and let her gradually take in some of the cool air that was gently wafting in. As soon as I felt she was ready to cope with the freezing temperature outside, I draped her arm over my shoulder and escorted her out. Then it came again, the same two words in an almost inaudible drawl, "Drink, sp—"

Two of my colleagues, who happened to be standing idle close by, managed to catch what the young woman was saying, and followed us outside to make light of it all. "Drink spiked? I don't think so. What a load of porkies!" said one of them, wagging a judgemental finger at her. Too far gone to even care that she wasn't being taken seriously, the young woman continued rolling her eyes around in her head as if she'd given up the will to live.

As far as my two colleagues were concerned, it was the young woman's own fault that she'd got herself in trouble. Bouncers are sometimes only too eager to sentence women in these situations, and find them guilty before they even have a shred of evidence. I, on the other hand, knew that there was some measure of truth in her muttering because I'd caught a stranger out of the corner of my eye, toying with her glass earlier on.

The clean air outside hadn't made any difference, and whatever drug was inside the young woman was now doing its worst. She suddenly began to shake uncontrollably, and with me no longer able to hold her up, she lost control of her legs and hit the pavement. A pitiful way to end the night perhaps, but she was one of the lucky ones: she, at least, would be waking up the next morning in her own bed.

VERBAL WARNING SIGNS

When it comes to keeping yourself safe in social situations, there are some important verbal warning signs to watch out for. Rushed dialogue probably means that a stranger doesn't have the time, or the inclination, to listen to you. Loud and forceful words are designed to disempower you. If the stranger isn't letting you answer questions, or finish sentences, then there are control issues there as well. And if his story doesn't hold – if there is so much as a hint of conflicting information – then you know that the stranger you are talking to has something to hide. If you put all this together, you end up with a stranger who has no interest in what you are saying, who is trying to take your power away, and who has a hidden agenda. For what possible reason could he be talking to you? Work that one out and you have cracked the verbal bully's code.

If you can't hear respect in a man's words, then find another.

"May I check your case, sir?" I asked a man one night as he waited to be searched. The man did a double take: he was usually the person handing out the orders. I tried to reassure him that my request was merely a formality, but he interrupted me before I could finish.

"Go ahead," he said, with calm hostility. "You seem rather tense. Why don't you relax a bit?" The man's voice was as smooth as oil, and equally sickly.

"Actually," I answered, "I'm feeling perfectly rela—" Again, I was cut dead.

"You see," he interjected, puffing himself up like a bellows about to fan, "when you take things easy, you do a much better job."

I opened my mouth to agree with him when he butted in again. "So don't get into a state. Don't worry your little head over things," he said, working himself up to a second wind. "What are your hobbies?"

"Well, I like martial a—" Cut off, yet again.

"I just ask," he continued, removing his diamante sunglasses and throwing me a haughty stare, "because I haven't seen you here before. You're new, aren't you?"

I had to hand it to the man: his drive to undermine wouldn't let up. I'd seen this type of bully so often before and had been challenged by the best of them. Through suave means or brutish, they'd never fail to use one-way dialogue as a weapon to overpower. I knew how to hold my own. Experience had taught me that there were only two ways of dealing with a verbal bully: interrupt the interrupter, or move away. Having no choice but to stay put – my job was to confront bullies and stop them from getting inside – I chose to play him at his own game and drown him out the next time I spoke. Anyway, it was time to show him that all his stalling tactics hadn't succeeded in distracting me from checking his case.

"I'd like you to move to the side and open your case – please," I commanded, talking over him.

Realizing that he no longer held the reins of power, the man's iron control crumbled, leaving exposed a molten core. Enraged, he threw open his case and pushed it under my nose. "There you are! See! No guns there!" he snarled.

At that moment, the manager of the place popped out for a quick smoke. When he saw who I was searching, he dived into a dark corner of the entrance and furiously waved me over. "Charly," he whispered, "you're not going to let him inside, are you?" The manager was usually a laid-back sort of chap, but had now become very nervous. "Not a chance," I replied under my breath. "The man won't let me finish a sentence. What I call a power stealer. Bad people."

"Good judgement call, Charly," said the manager, tiptoeing his way back inside. "We barred him a few weeks back. Drugs baron. Dangerous. Keep him busy while I go and call the police."

THE CHAIN OF EVENTS

An oft-repeated line is that an attack comes out of nowhere. This couldn't be further from the truth: there is always a chain of events leading up to an attack. If an attacker strikes you by surprise, it means that you haven't been paying attention; it means that you have only noticed the last stage in the chain of events – the attack. It also means that you have been oblivious to everything that has led up to that point. Warning signs are always there to help you stay out of trouble. The buck rests with you to notice them.

A stranglehold comes after your personal space has been invaded, which comes after a verbal interchange, which comes after an initial approach, which comes after you have been singled out. Let us look at all that the other way round. You have been singled out by an attacker, who then approaches you, talks to you, invades your personal space, and finally attacks you. There are more stages taking place here than you might suspect – each one is a link in a chain. If you deal with the earliest link in the chain, your chances of survival are much greater because with each link, your attacker is getting closer. Leaving things until the last link in the chain could mean disaster. So be aware of people watching you. Notice any interest you might be attracting whenever you are out clubbing, or at a bus stop, or anywhere in a public place. This is the first warning sign to look out for. Think of yourself as the bird that catches the worm – early.

A young woman was violated one night and sought retribution for the injustice. After only five minutes with a stranger on the dance floor, he indecently assaulted her – she was spitting venom. She tugged at my shirt

sleeve and said that if I didn't throw her abuser out, she'd do it herself. I explained that she'd have to come with me to identify the man, and that before I could confront him, I needed the full story. It went something like this: the first time she saw the stranger, he was harassing another woman on the dance floor. He grabbed the woman's hand, but she resisted and pulled away. She then saw the stranger yank the woman back towards him and put his arms around her. The woman fought to break free, and once out of the stranger's clutches, expressed her refusal to spend one more moment with him on the dance floor. It was then that he slid his hand up her skirt, just to spite her.

The young woman stopped her account. Reliving the sordid drama of it all was more than she could stand, and she became hysterical. "I wanna f—g skin the a—e alive! Let me at him!" she ranted, fingernails poised as if she were already flaying her abuser to shreds. She launched herself towards the dance floor to hunt down her attacker, but it was plain that she was in no mood to be rational, and that settling a score using violence would probably not work out in her favour. I grabbed her in a tight bear hug and bundled her, kicking and screaming, into the security room nearby.

It didn't take long for her rage to die down. With the dance floor out of sight, and her abuser nowhere near striking distance, the young woman flopped into an armchair, buried her face in her hands, and wept. As tears of anger flowed, the emotional pain of her assault began to kick in. She turned her attention away from the dance floor, and settled long enough to tell me the second part of her story. It went something like this: shortly after the woman she'd seen being assaulted left, the stranger approached her. While she didn't like the look of the man, she felt sure that she'd probably be alright – one dance couldn't hurt, after all. But no sooner had they started dancing than he began to get a little too familiar with her as well. He pressed himself so closely against her that she could feel his sweat. She shoved him off, told him to get lost, and turned to walk away. Unable to cope with the rejection, the stranger repeated his earlier indiscretion and slipped his hand somewhere it shouldn't have been.

That was the last word from the young woman. An overwhelming grief enveloped her like a dark shroud, and she went to silence. She cradled her stomach and rocked herself as if nursing a deep wound. The whole wretched affair deeply saddened me. I hated seeing women abused in this way. The kind of damage inflicted by this type of assault was always so much more than skin deep.

Weary and solemn, I pulled up a stool and sat facing the young woman as she cried. Like a priest in a confession box, all I could do was listen. Knowing that I couldn't undo her violation, I felt moved to say something that might prevent it ever happening again. When I felt she was ready to see the part she'd played in bringing it about, I gently held her face in my hands and asked, "At what point in this sorry tale did you not see trouble coming?" I never did get my answer.

Chapter Two

SOME WISDOM FOR THE STREET

DARK ALLEYS

Dark alleys are for those who can see in the dark. Avoid them, always. It is no defeat to choose a way home that is well lit. If your visibility is compromised in any way, you won't be able to see trouble coming. Defending blind is your worst case scenario.

Some women argue that this is a free world we live in, and that being a truly liberated woman is about being able to go where you please, and do what you want. They also say that not being controlled by the threat of danger is a matter of principle. I would answer that survival is a matter of principle as well. It is really just a question of priority: being right, or staying safe.

I said goodnight to a young woman just as we were closing. She was tired and worse for wear and, in spite of me insisting that she get a taxi home, she assured me that she was quite capable of walking. Home was not that far after all, and anyway, she felt quite safe in the area as she was a local girl.
I felt uneasy about this, and repeated that it would be prudent for her to catch a cab – I knew of a reliable company that could take her home. She was adamant that no harm would come to her. "Nothing ever happens to me!" she stated as she headed out to the street.
I never saw the young woman again, but a colleague of mine, who knew her, told me the next week that she'd been attacked that night on her way home. She'd opted for a fast route back; a narrow shortcut that was unlit. A thug, who'd been waiting in the shadows to rob someone, had tripped

her up, beaten her to within an inch of her life, and taken off with her handbag. The next thing the young woman saw were the faces of her family peering over her as she lay recovering in a hospital bed. Sometimes the shortest route home is the longest.

RUMBLING THE STREET ATTACKER

It is amazing just how much dark energy you can fend off, if you are sharp enough to see it approach. I heard a line once that said the devil can never creep up on you if you see him coming. There is a lot of truth in that. Not once, in all my time as a bouncer, did I ever see an attacker successfully jump someone who saw them approach. If you rumble a street thug and spot him early, you will cut out nearly all danger in one swoop. I hear people pay lip service to this strategy. So many say they are vigilant when out and about, but very few ever are. A great pity, because catching out the devil is so much easier than you would imagine. It is often a question of spotting the obvious: that the devil's best work is done right under your very nose.

As a woman, you have a distinct advantage over a man in seeing an attacker coming. The pre-attack phase between a man and a woman is often much longer, and more drawn out, than that between two men. If an attacker isn't after your wallet, he will be following you to violate you physically. If you are out alone late at night and a stranger approaches with this intention in mind, he must remove you from where you are – unless there is no chance that he can be seen. This stage will almost always involve some dialogue.

So, two pre-attack stages emerge: approach and dialogue. Becoming aware of these two stages can greatly increase your chances of survival – most attackers can be seen off at this point. You will need to be open to making a decision and acting on it quickly, though, as the pre-attack phase can happen in a heartbeat. Learning to identify the stages involved in the pre-attack phase really levels the playing field.

There was always a risk on the doors that someone you threw out might

decide to wait for you outside to settle a score later on as you left. A few of my colleagues did have some serious run-ins with clubbers they'd ejected. Lowlifes with murder in mind would sometimes hover outside in the dark, and wait to savage them after we'd closed. My colleagues so often did something that I considered extraordinary: they'd walk straight out at the end of the night with absolutely no care, or regard, for their safety. No checking to see who might be outside; no bothering about any potential thugs wanting retribution for having been slung out. It was all a bit of an enigma.

As a result of this false sense of security, some of the men I worked with met with some very nasty injuries. I did warn them, though. Before they left each night, I'd remind them to watch their backs. My advice fell on deaf ears, and they'd all wander out through the doors in what I call "code oblivious". I gave up in the end.

My experience was very different to theirs. At the end of each night, I'd make a point of scanning the area outside each venue as I left it. During my entire time on the doors, I only ever had one problem with a clubber harbouring a grudge for having been shown the door. I'd had to throw out a young woman early one night because she'd been drinking heavily, and was beginning to challenge other female clubbers to a punch-up. No sooner had I got her outside than she phoned her boyfriend to tell him what had happened. She was bitter that she'd been ejected, but I was confident that she'd calm down, eventually. I didn't give the matter another thought until I was leaving. As I walked out into the night after we'd finished for the evening, I gave the area my usual once-over to make sure I was safe, and there she was, still in the same place leaning over one of the metal barriers where I'd left her – only now she was with her boyfriend. The two of them were punching the air in my direction and spitting obscenities from just yards away. Cursing through gnashing teeth and with a broken bottle in hand, the boyfriend charged towards me with his girlfriend in tow. Still only a short distance away from the front door, I turned and raced to get back inside. The pair was hot on my heels and chased me there, but having the advantage of a few seconds, I made it to the door in time and quickly slammed it shut, clipping their noses in the process. With injury now added to fury, the pair began hurling themselves bodily against the front door like a couple of Rottweilers trying to weaken a fence.

As I quietly left by the back exit, I could still hear their fists and feet pounding at the door. I was shaken about the night's events, not because *of what happened, but because of what might have happened.*

HOOKS

A hook is any strategy, or distraction, an attacker uses to bring him close enough to harm you. It usually starts as a question. "Can you tell me the time?" or "Can you tell me the way to —" You look down at your watch to see what time it is, or you turn your head around to point out directions, and before you know where you are, your bag has been stolen – or worse. When out and about, treat any question from a stranger as a hook designed to reel you in. Ignore it; don't get sucked in. Anyway, hooks are for fish.

Men were often curious about female bouncers. I'd often be at the receiving end of a barrage of personal questions that were designed to draw me in. I was different from the women they knew and they'd press me for details about my life. Whenever this happened, I'd stonewall them. I'd flat out blank any questions coming my way, and just keep walking. Often, when it was clear that I wasn't playing ball, the questions grew more persistent. When they did, I'd give my questioners a meaningless brush-off line – these had a way of stopping any conversation dead in its tracks.
One night, a man asked me if I enjoyed being a female bouncer – he was just chucking me a line to see if I'd bite. "Toad in the hole!" I shrieked, pointing at his feet. Before he could trot out another question, I was on the other side of the club downing a lime and lemonade.

SCANNING

When out in public, your safety zone extends as far as your eye can see. As you walk, get used to scanning as often as you can. Scan your immediate area, but like a lion that keeps an eye out for any potential danger on the horizon, also take in the world at a greater distance. On the street, you need to be watching near, as well as far, to pre-empt the patter of danger's feet.

I used to amuse myself on quiet nights watching people approach the front door from a distance. From there, it was ever so easy to see who was walking in a straight line, and who wasn't. One night, an intoxicated man was making painfully slow progress towards the front door from a quarter of a mile away. With his top half leaning one way, and his bottom half leaning the other, he set a straight course for the front door – on the diagonal. As if an invisible tightrope were pulling him to centre, he veered back on course with every few steps. He was only yards from the front door when he did a three hundred and sixty degree sway, without falling over. The man steadied himself, clapped his outstretched hands together in front of him, and did a wobbly tango all the way to the front door. "Can I come in, miss?" he asked. "Not tonight, sir," I said.

ATTACKERS WITH KNIVES

A practical tip on knife culture is that an attacker who displays the knife he is threatening you with is generally less likely to use it – he is just trying to scare you into submission. An attacker is much more likely to use a knife if he has it hidden. If you find yourself alone on an empty street and a stranger approaches, make sure you can see both his hands. The street predator with a knife is a bit like a poker player: he never puts all his cards on the table.

There are two reasons why a man with a knife will attack you: he will either be after your wallet, or his intention will be to hurt you physically. With the first one, you have two things on your side: distance, and your wallet. Often, the knife attacker after your money doesn't close the gap between you completely: he will threaten you with a knife from a small distance away. This gives you enough space to do one vital thing: show him your wallet, and throw it. Make sure that it lands behind him. Remember, it is your money he wants, so he will turn around and race to pick it up. This widens the gap between you, giving you a few seconds to get away.

The second reason a man with a knife will attack will be to rape you, kill you, or both. The knife attacker who intends to do either of these, or both, will almost certainly grab you from behind – most street attacks on women happen this way. Unfortunately, this means that your advantage of distance will probably be gone. If it has, you will just have to go with the flow and wait for an opportunity to defend. There will be one – there always is. If you are lucky enough to see an attack coming from ahead, then honour the golden rule of distance and keep as much space as possible between you. If there is any large object close to hand – a shopping trolley for example – push it in between you and the attacker. Throw anything big you can get your hands on to stop the attacker from closing the gap.

Your most important defence against a knife attack is, as with any other, your ability to notice. So when you are out alone, pay close attention to the space all around you. Study your surroundings, and always keep an ear to the ground. While it is impossible to see someone creeping up behind you, you can hear them, if you stay alert.

As I stood at the bar ordering a soft drink, I tried to look the part of a serial clubber instead of an undercover bouncer. Management at the north London club had implemented stiff measures to combat drug trafficking – as well as any other illegal goings-on. I was the newest kid on the security block, and was chosen to patrol the dance floor that night in plain clothes.

It didn't take long for a stranger on the prowl to sidle up. "Wanna drink, babe?" he asked, presumptuously.

I humoured him and strung him along for a while to find out more. There was something shady about the man; something that I felt warranted a closer look. "I'll have an apple juice, please," I answered. As he reached inside his pocket for some money, a small object fell on the floor. I bent down to pick up what looked like a knife. "I think this is yours," I said.

"Cheers, babe," he answered, slipping it back into his pocket. "That's me backup." I was intrigued and asked him to explain what he meant. "It's me little safety net, is me flick knife!" he bragged.

The man was so eager to impress that he continued, quite openly, to enlighten me on the virtues of concealing a knife. "Should any t—r give me any trouble, I can spring the blade out while it's still in me pocket and stick 'im one quickly!"

I gulped down my apple juice, made my excuses, and hurried to the ladies' room to alert my colleagues of the situation. In a matter of minutes, the man found himself across the road waiting for a night bus home, without his knife. That was my introduction to knife culture on the street – straight from the horse's mouth.

CODE YELLOW

Visualizing colour is a tool that can help you stay safe on the street. You can use it as a trigger to switch you into an appropriate mood, depending on where you are. Let me explain: when you are at home, or visiting friends, you are safe enough to be in what is called a "code white" frame of mind. White symbolizes purity, so when you imagine yourself to be in a "code white" mood, you can afford to relax and let your guard down; you can go out into the garden and smell the roses without having to watch your back. But when you head out to the street, remember to switch from a "code white", to a "code yellow" frame of mind. Yellow stands for illumination. Like the sun, it casts light over everything. When you are in "code yellow", there isn't anything that you can't see; nothing hidden, or in shadow, can remain in darkness so there are no surprises. You will see the street thug before he sees you. If you are still in "code white", you won't see him at all. Ignorance isn't bliss.

I noticed as a bouncer that nightclubs were brimming with people in "code white". That was why there was always so much trouble in these places: nobody ever noticed anything.

It was a sad day when I was told that David wasn't going to be the head doorman anymore at the east London club I was working at. I was the only female out of five of us manning the doors, and as far as most of my colleagues were concerned, I was a waste of space. David thought otherwise: he trusted me and told me so. The man thought so highly of me in fact, that he gave me the first real crack of the whip I'd ever had on the doors. David's last night springs to mind.

It was New Year's Eve, and twice as many people as usual had turned up. We were all standing outside just after we'd opened up, when David suddenly called us all over to one side. "Now look you guys, this is going to be a busy one. I need two of you out here managing the punters as they come in, and I need two of you inside." My colleagues shoved me sideways as they pushed in to hear more. "Tim and Stuart, out here with me. Charly and Alex, inside."

I groaned. How I wished that for once, I'd been able to work with someone else. I dreaded being paired up with Alex: he was bad at his job and was always oblivious to what was going on around him. Most of all, he was arrogant. My face must have given me away. "Alex, hold up a minute before you disappear," said David, reading my mind. "I want Charly to be in charge inside. Any questions, ask her."

Alex, who never normally paid attention to anything, stood bolt upright with indignation. "Why are you putting her in charge? I've been here longer!" he whined.

"Because she watches. She keeps her eyes peeled," answered David, pointing two fingers at his eyes. "She also has the most presence." Alex swore under his breath and walked inside behind me.

That evening proved to be the club's first trouble-free New Year's Eve bash on record. A few heated arguments had erupted, but nothing you could worry about. Shortly before leaving, I caught up with David at the bar. I said a last goodbye and let him know he'd be missed. David was such a rare breed because he didn't give a fig about what sex you were as a bouncer. To him, all that mattered was performance.

With a heavy heart, I headed for the exit. I was three paces from the door when David swung round, raised his whisky glass, and with a proud grin shouted, "I had you out for a 'yellow' from the start, Charly!"

"Is that 'yellow' for coward?" I asked.

"Nah. 'Yellow' for switched on!" he replied.

WINGSPAN

When you close down physically, you are making yourself less than you are – this is the opposite of standing in your power. Making yourself any less than you are, on any level, isn't the way to go when it comes to your personal safety. Next time you are on a bus or a train, notice the body language of other women. Watch how a woman sits down next to a stranger: does she expand and take up more space, or does she contract? Most women will try to occupy as little space as possible when they are in the company of people they don't know. The problem with this is that when you physically shrink in the presence of a stranger, you are showing him submission. And if that stranger happens to be a potential attacker, then you are giving him the green light.

To break this unconscious pattern, you must give yourself permission to take whatever physical space you need to feel comfortable and safe. You also need to become aware of your behaviour when you are out and about. As you walk down a street, for example, notice the movement of your head. When a man approaches you, pay close attention to whether or not you lower your head. Dipping your head, even slightly, is a primal statement that any male passer-by will register subliminally – it reinforces gender pecking order. It took me years to catch myself doing this, and once I had, I assumed that I was doing it with everyone. But one day, I was walking down a street and a woman passed me. I didn't drop my head – even slightly. This aspect of body language is subtle, but it can teach you volumes about what is really going on inside you. I call it the shrinking and lowering behaviour pattern that many women unconsciously internalize.

Not giving away your power has everything to do with using all of your physical space – your wingspan – and pulling up physically. When it comes to your wingspan, size is *everything*. The more space you claim, and the taller you walk, the less likely a street thug will be to see you as bait. A good exercise to practise to help you break the shrinking and lowering pattern, is to find a quiet spot at home where you won't be disturbed. Stand in the middle of the room and stretch out your arms as wide as comfort will allow. Take in all of the space around you and trace an invisible line, upwards and outwards. Close your eyes, and feel as if your arms are growing – they are so long that you can touch the walls. Feel the power of that stretch – it is your stretch. That distance is your wingspan. It is the distance that *no* person should ever penetrate without your permission.

No animal would dare to overstep the mark where spatial boundaries are concerned. Animals are highly respectful of each other's space. There are only two reasons why two animals of the opposite sex will invade each other's wingspan: one is to attack, the other is to procreate. That should give you plenty to think about when it comes to deciding whom to let near, and how close they should get.

Developing a rock solid wingspan starts with becoming conscious of the space that surrounds you. Take a look around: all that space that you see seems empty, but it is actually filled with sounds, smells, and sights that travel through it, and give you vital information about your safety. Think of the emptiness around you as an invisible blanket; a protective layer rather like the atmosphere around the earth. A powerful visualization to do to connect with your wingspan is to imagine that it is physically concrete and tangible. Try to imagine what it looks like. Is it a colour? Does it have a shape? Has it got a name? After a while, you will begin to sense an energetic force around you that people will register unknowingly. Once you have built your wingspan, stand back and watch the world respond.

On the most hectic nights it was a given that I'd get pushed and shoved every which way. At these times, I often wondered if there was anything I could do to stop myself from getting squashed to a pulp. I already knew, in theory, what being conscious of a wingspan could achieve where personal space was concerned. As I headed out to work one night, it dawned on me that patrolling the busiest of dance floors would be an ideal opportunity to clearly sense my wingspan, and see what it could do in practice.

I walked through the front door of an east London nightclub and was greeted by a tetchy head doorman. The atmosphere outside the place was already electric enough with the voices of regulars getting into full swing, but the atmosphere inside was a swing and a punch away from uproar – peak time ravers, hostile clubbers fighting for space, and a security team itching to use unreasonable force. This was the perfect setting to work on keeping both my physical, and invisible, boundaries intact.

With purpose in my step, I made my way inside. Before I'd even reached my usual position by the dance floor, my wingspan was in place. Like a soldier going into battle, my full metal jacket of invisible power had been activated. I knew what colour it was, how thick it felt, and what it was made of. I could feel the presence of this energetic cocoon so vividly, that it was as if my physical body had stretched five feet in all directions.

I stood keeping an eagle eye over a corner of the dance floor and noticed something odd: a semicircle of space started to open up in front of me. All the clubbers, quite unconsciously, were dancing around me about five feet away, but no closer. For the entire time I was patrolling that part of the dance floor, an invisible wall kept them at that fixed distance. Later on that night as I patrolled other dance floors, the same thing happened. A layer of empty space would always surround me no matter where I stood.

I spent the next few weeks trying to explain it all. Bouncers, I reasoned, weren't always the most approachable of types – perhaps people were avoiding me. But after months of seeing how differently clubbers reacted to me once I had a strong sense of my wingspan, I eventually made the connection. And very pleased I was to have made it: it not only reinforced the importance of walking tall and fat, it also took my understanding of how the physical can be affected by the invisible, to a new level.

CREATING A FENCE

A fence is a powerful physical statement that tells someone to keep their distance. If you find yourself in a public place and a stranger approaches who you wish wouldn't, put your arms straight up in front of you, with palms facing outward. Even if you feel silly doing it, have a go – the reaction you will get will be worth it. You might startle a few people when your fence goes up, but so what? You are exploring the effectiveness of a physical defence, and the only way to see what it can do is to act it out.

Creating a fence to keep people at a safe distance is body language at its most direct. People will very quickly get your drift, often without you having to say a word. It is a very handy way to make a point.

The right time to create a fence is whenever you feel a need to. If you think about it, honestly, how many times have you felt spatially violated? Get a pen and paper and try to recall as many incidents as you can where a man got too close, and where you felt powerless to change that. Ask yourself why it was that you allowed this to happen. Ask yourself why you didn't honour your right as a human being to preserve your personal boundary. Also think about how you experience distance. Next time you are talking to a stranger, observe the body language taking place between you: are you both getting closer, and if so, just who is closing the gap?

Putting up a fence teaches you to be comfortable with taking the initiative. When you take the initiative, you are standing in your power. Understand that with all woman-to-man interaction, there are only two ways you can go as far as initiative is concerned: either *you* are taking it, or *he* is. If you haven't put up a barrier to protect yourself when an intruder oversteps the mark, you have allowed the intruder to set the pace. And if that happens, then you aren't keeping potential danger out, you are inviting it in.

It was standard nightclub policy to stop people coming in two hours before closing time. One night, just as I was about to shut the front door, a young man ran towards me and begged me to let him in. He argued that he'd already been inside earlier on with friends, and felt it only right that he should be allowed back in.

I was quick to fill him in on some nightclub protocol and explained that after midnight, no one was allowed in – irrespective of whether they'd already been inside or not. He nodded sulkily and wandered off – I thought that would be an end of it. The young man had other ideas: he loitered outside in the dark near the entrance, hoping for a chance to try and bulldoze his way back in. I ignored him and stood outside guarding the front door like a she wolf – his only way in, was out.

Seeing no chance of sneaking past me unnoticed, he cast all caution to the winds, took a running jump, and made a headlong rush for the door. With only six feet between us, I shot my arms up, stood as solid as an oak, and braced myself for impact. The young tearaway crashed into my uplifted palms, bounced off, and staggered backwards into the middle of the road, landing on his backside. The last thing I remember is of him being helped to his feet by a frail, elderly lady who happened to be passing by. Humiliated at having been overpowered by one woman, and embarrassed at being rescued by another, he scowled as he stood up, and ran to the nearest taxi rank to wait for a ride home. Never "de-fence" yourself if trouble comes a-visiting. Call everyone's bluff and stand your ground – that's most of the battle won.

SPACE INVADERS

A space invader is anyone who invades your personal space and makes you feel uncomfortable. Your personal space can be any distance from you – it is up to you. If a man penetrates your personal boundary, take action and immediately re-establish it. If he follows you and moves in again, use this as valuable information – it tells you all about the person you are with. It tells you that the sacred boundary you have just set up has been violated. If this happens more than once, then not only is your boundary being disrespected, it is being trashed. Give all space invaders the widest berth, and understand that they are not waiting to be asked to come closer: they are forcing closeness *uninvited.*

All space invaders use their physical presence to overpower you. Some of them do this unconsciously, while others are very aware of closing an unacceptable gap. Space invaders, as a bunch, are an unsubtle lot. They are not remotely bothered about disregarding any needs you might have, because they are far more interested in their own. The law of reciprocity dictates that you should only care about someone if they care about you. If any care that you have so kindly bestowed isn't returned, then you are energetically out of pocket. Don't give a space invader's feelings a second thought – you are *not* an energetic charity. Be bold in both action and word, and clearly define your boundary. Spell it all out, just as if you were talking to someone who didn't speak a word of English. I am afraid that nothing less will make the slightest dent.

A colleague I worked with on the doors would insist on getting too close every time he spoke to me. One quiet night while keeping an eye on the front door shortly before closing time, we had little to do and were running out of ways to wax lyrical about the silvery moon above. To break, what I considered to be a welcome silence, my colleague thought it a plum idea to share some personal, heroic experiences of his time on the doors. As he did so, he walked so close to me that I could feel his breath on my cheek. In order to re-establish my personal space, I swapped places with him and shimmied back to where he'd been standing only moments earlier, but the man just followed me. I walked back a second time to where he'd moved from, in the hope that he'd take the hint and stay an acceptable distance away, but he didn't. He was oblivious to my efforts to maintain personal space, and so engrossed in relating every single spat he'd ever had as a bouncer, that he closed the gap yet again. I took the bull by the horns and confronted him. I pointed out that I could hear him quite well enough from where he was, and that I needed some distance – being stalked from only feet away was unacceptable. The directness of my demand killed his rambling, and for a while, he honoured my wishes. Later on, though, our exasperating game of tag resumed. Unable to resist impressing me with the conclusion of his vainglorious adventures, he inched closer again. Just as he was about to close any gap left, I put my hands on my hips, stuck out my elbows, and gave him the sharp end of them in his ribs as he closed in.

Mid-waffle, he turned and strolled back to where he should have been in the first place. On some level, he must have got the message because he remained at a comfortable distance from me for the rest of the night. Next time a space invader gets too close, try giving him the elbow – it works a treat.

COMMITTING

Whether you are embroiled in a bit of verbal sparring, or whether you find yourself in a physical confrontation, try to avoid overly committing to either an opinion, or a strike. The more energy you invest in any action, the harder it is to alter its course. So commit to winning, and to staying safe, but be prepared to chop and change on the way to doing this. Not committing too heavily keeps you just ahead of the game – should the rules suddenly change.

Two men on a dance floor were both vying for the same woman. Voices rose, stances began to square up, and in no time, the pre-fight stage of a violent episode was under way. As they moved closer, each man's commitment to destroy the other increased with every step. Earlier on, either one could have walked away with some semblance of dignity. Now, it was too late for either to step down, even if they'd wanted to. And all this over a woman who'd long gone.

Chapter Three

SIFTING THE ANGELS FROM THE DEMONS

DARK ENERGY

There is a reliable way to spot one of Darth Vader's cronies whenever you are out and about. There is one blinding trademark, one common denominator that all those working for the dark side share: they are all immediate. Whether they are after your wallet or your life force, they will need it on the "hurry, hurry". If you think about it, the street thug who threatens you for your wallet wants it now. Have you ever heard of a mugger telling his victim to take their time handing it over? Better still, he will pop around the corner for a coffee while they make up their mind. The rapist who attacks you while you walk home alone is after your life force. I can't remember ever hearing of an attacker threatening to rape a woman "sometime whenever". If you are going to be violated, it will happen *now*.

In any social situation, if you feel you are being pressured into things, even a tad, slow down. Take your time, and don't be rushed. Pad things out as much as circumstance will allow. The one thing that all those operating from the dark side will not do, is wait. So give them the runaround. Find the absolute slowest boat to China, jump aboard, and travel with all recommended types on the "slowly, slowly".

Dark energy isn't lit as it has no light of its own. Dark energy isn't conscious as it doesn't know what it is. Dark energy is a rudderless ship that will be led this way and that because it has no centre.

Three of us were outside manning the front door late one night, when a

garbled message came over our radios from a colleague at the back exit.
"Guys, I've just kicked out some a—e. Make sure he doesn't get back in at
the front!"

Unfortunately for us, our colleague at the back exit failed to tell us what
the man he'd just ejected looked like. Before we had a chance to find out,
the troublemaker had raced round to the entrance, grabbed a metal
rubbish bin, and hurled it at us. The bin missed. Enraged that he hadn't
inflicted any damage, the young thug charged towards us to finish the job.

The three of us were a good team – almost telepathic. As soon as the
young thug was within striking distance, we grabbed him and pulled him
to the ground without even exchanging a word. As we wrestled to keep him
there, one of my colleagues leant over and muttered under his breath, "I
bet you'd rather be at home in Canary Wharf right now, Charly."

How, in all of creation, anyone could have heard this quiet aside amid all
the commotion, was something utterly beyond us. Incredibly, though, our
attacker did hear it. "I'm gonna f—g bomb Canary Wharf! You're gonna
die, you bitch!" he yelled, trying to claw and kick his way free. "I have
friends who can arrange it!" We froze. Years on the doors had taught us
the difference between an empty threat and a serious one. We made eye
contact, and at the count of three hauled the young thug into the security
room so fast he didn't even have time to resist.

Now out of public view, we felt sure we would be able to take things to the
next level, but as soon as the security room door slammed shut, the young
thug wriggled free and was up swinging punches before we could restrain
him. We all dropped on top of him at the same time and, with the three of
us spread all over him like a tent, we finally had control. The young thug,
who was now unable to move and only just able to breathe, conceded
defeat. After ten minutes in a one-against-three he had no more energy left
to hit out. He did, however, have enough energy left to wage war verbally
and his poison continued. "I'll have you all killed! You stinking, rotten
westerners! Everything I've been told is true: you're all f—g evil and must
be f—g wiped out!"

We had just never seen this level of darkness before. Threats of violence,
though, have no power over three minds that have processed and
transcended all inner demons. Without speaking, we closed in and
surrounded the young thug like three penguins shielding themselves from
an arctic wind. We stood as silent witnesses to all of the young coward's
darkest inner machinations. We gave him all the space he needed to spit
out whatever evil grandiosity he cared to share, and we let him run this

course unbridled.

Now too hoarse to shout, the young thug's anger slowly trailed off, and with only the last embers of his rage left, he settled. We picked him up off the floor and sat him down. An air of resignation swept through him as if some invisible, malevolent hand had reached down, punctured his skull, and switched him off. He took a deep breath, lowered his head, and quietly prayed.

When the police arrived he offered no resistance as they cuffed him and carted him off. As I watched him leave, it occurred to me that he had no idea who he was. He had no sense of self to tell him why he thought the things he did. His inner voice had been lost, and outsiders had replaced it with dark things that had him beating to the sound of their drum, rather than to the sound of his own.

THE LAW OF ATTRACTION

The universal law of attraction is an amazing thing. It never wavers and is constant – no exceptions. Whatever thought form or action you put out will fly back at you boomerang-style. On that basis, never physically or mentally put out anything, unless you are quite happy for it to come racing back.

A good exercise to do to help you gauge whether or not you belong somewhere, is to sit quietly and visualize the location you are going to, and mark it out of ten – energetically. Where do you think it is on that scale, with zero for black, dark energy, and ten for balanced, bright, and centred energy? Spend a few moments doing this whenever you head out to a public place – your mind's eye can be trusted. Any number your inner vision comes up with is a reliable guide for whether or not you are energetically matched for a place. When I am out and about, I visualize my way around like this all the time. It enables me to decide whether to bolt, or hang around.

While I was guarding the front door alone one night, a clubber, with cigarette and drink in hand, staggered outside for some fresh air. "God,

*it's so smoky in there," he moaned, half choking. "Can't you do something
to clear the air inside? I can't breathe in that place!"*
*I pointed out to the man that if he was that bothered about the smoke,
perhaps he should leave. He threw me a quizzical stare, lit another
cigarette, and croaked, "Can't you do anything at all? I'm asthmatic!"*
Dark energy always finds its own level.

READING INVISIBLE ENERGY

All human beings project a stream of invisible energy, all of the time. This
electromagnetic charge travels towards you in pulses from what is sometimes
referred to as the luminous, or energetic body. Most people can't see the
energetic body, but if you open to the subtle, you will eventually be able to
sense it and feel other people's luminous bodies hitting yours. The energetic
bodies of those holding a lot of darkness stand out. If you pass someone and
feel something malevolent about them, you are almost certainly responding to
something unpleasant contained within their energy body. All of our physical,
mental, and emotional make-up, is stored within the luminous body as an
imprint – the reason why those who carry a dark inner force leave a trail of dull,
stagnant energy behind them.

If you can become adept at spotting people's dark trails, you will have access to
something very special: the ability to see the invisible. I use this tracking
system all the time. Any hint of a bad, luminous body odour and I will
respectfully keep my distance. As you go about your day, try and feel people's
energetic bodies. As people pass you by, try and sense their energetic bodies
tapping yours; see if you can register how heavy or light they feel. Also notice
whether they feel thin, or stretched. A useful way to gauge someone's
luminous body is to imagine it as a colour. Generally, the darker the colour in
your mind's eye the more negativity that person will be holding. Have a blast,
but mostly, honour whatever comes.

*A man I'd never seen before walked in through the doors one night, and I
knew he'd be trouble. An energetic haze surrounded him like a cloud of
soot. As he approached, I felt as if I were being weighted down – a sure
sign of someone's inner darkness. As he swaggered past on his way to the
bar, my skin prickled as if I'd been stung by tiny invisible darts.*

I hesitated before saying anything because this was my first shift at a new venue. I didn't know the men I was working with, or how they would react to one of their team using inner vision to weed out troublemakers. In the interests of keeping the peace, I decided to express my doubts – in a language they would understand. "Guys, that one will be a problem. I'd put money on it."

My colleagues, who recognized the man as a regular, were quite happy for him to waltz in unchecked. They'd become complacent where he was concerned and cordially waved him in. "Charly, he's what we call one of our 'respectable' regulars," said one of them, ushering in another regular with a regal flick of his hand. "No need to worry. He's kosher. You'll get to know who all the troublemakers are soon enough."

I was quietly confident. I was also quite content being the only one who had any real insight into the truth of the matter. I knew that the man would disrespect my colleagues' trust at some point later on, even if they didn't. Anyway, I told myself, the truth would out sooner or later. As it happened, it turned out to be sooner. Only an hour after I'd voiced my concern, the message came over my radio that a fight had started. I raced from my station at the dance floor and got to the scene to find our "respectable" regular knocking seven bells out of a member of staff at the bar. The two were locked in an untidy scrum on the floor. I later found out that the "respectable" regular had had a score to settle with one of the barmen – it was this energy that I'd felt as he'd entered.

At the end of the night, while I was keeping an eye on the front door, my colleagues rather sheepishly sidled up wanting to know more about how I'd read the situation so accurately. I politely made my excuses, and wandered back inside. My colleagues were a friendly bunch, but there was no answer I could possibly give that would make any sense to them. People who believe only in what they can see will never acknowledge the invisible – they're not ready to. And no good can ever come from trying to explain it to them. It's a sacred thing to be able to see the invisible. When you see things that others can't, be a witness to truth, but keep it to yourself.

HOW TO JUDGE SOMEONE

If you want to get the true measure of people, don't listen to what they say, watch what they do. Don't be taken in with what a man tells you he feels, thinks, or knows – respect is a *behaviour*. Hold this truth close whenever you judge the world. It enables you to see beneath the veil, and sense the real motive behind a smile.

Rely only on your own assessment of someone when you judge them. If others tell you that someone is nice, wait and find out the truth of this for yourself. Suspend your information, and find out how nice that person is first-hand. You will be surprised at how much your opinion can vary from someone else's. A girlfriend tells you that a man she met recently at a party would be just perfect for you – check it out for yourself. Don't be influenced by what she says. Blind dates hardly ever work – for good reason.

A young woman, with her back to the wall, was being smooth-talked by a stranger. They'd only just met and I watched the two flirting and exchanging sweet nothings for a while – the scene was not unfamiliar. The young woman seemed to be open and responsive to her admirer's charms: she laughed in all the right places and, flattered by his attention, allowed the man to get closer physically. The young woman had, perhaps, not judged her suitor's character accurately: every chance he got, he'd look away and scan his surroundings. He wouldn't listen to her, or look at her for more than a few seconds before shifting a roving eye towards the dance floor in search of either more women, or other dominant males. The man's insincerity was lost on the young woman, who swooned for another couple of hours.

Later that evening, I wished them well as they left the club – the rest of the night would unfold as it would for them. All I can say is that the man in question was a regular who would be back the following week to find another plaything. As for the young woman, she also returned to the club some weeks later, but only to dance. Determined to put bad times behind her, and eager to move on, she greeted me with a sad smile and despairing eyes. The night she'd spent with the stranger had been one of crippling disappointment, for while she'd been looking to make a connection, he hadn't.

There had been warning signs that the stranger's intentions weren't serious. Had the young woman focussed, not on what her suitor was saying, but on everything he was doing, she might have guessed that they

were not well matched, and saved herself a lot of heartache.
Keeping yourself safe is about protecting all of you. Your mind, body, and
spirit are all vulnerable to attack. If you hurt one, you very likely hurt them
all.

LISTENING

Street thugs abound and often use charm to reel you in. The important thing is
to be able to blow their cover; to be able to spot the deception behind the words.
For that, you really need to fine-tune your listening skills and learn to listen
intensely. The more you practise this, the more you will be able to sense
whether someone is well meaning or not – irrespective of the words they are
using. I knew a blind man once: you could never lie to him – it would be foolish
to even try. He would sometimes hear the intention behind my words even
before I knew what it was. "All that glitters isn't gold," he used to tell me. I
asked him once if he found not being able to see gold a major handicap. "Not
really," he replied. "I can see so much more with my ears. Anyway," he
whispered, as if letting me in on a secret, "the answers are always blowing in
the wind."

A doe in the woods listens carefully for the faintest sound, and before even a
hint of danger manifests, will hear a twig snap somewhere it shouldn't and will
be off. One's senses aren't set: they can be developed with practice. A powerful
exercise to help your listening skills grow by leaps and bounds, is to practise
listening to noises and sounds with a blindfold on – cut out your vision. The
results will amaze you. When you hear the sound of an engine starting, for
example, register the sound of it, and without any judgement or comment, say
inwardly to yourself, "Car." After a while, move on to something harder: see if
you can hear the sound of your own heartbeat. Once you can do that, you will
be able to hear your way out of almost any kind of trouble.

I'd always assumed that a noisy dance floor would be the last place where
I could sharpen my listening skills – one incident proved me wrong. I was

stationed at the corner of a packed dance floor one night, when my ears picked up the faint, but incongruous noise of someone coughing. This wasn't normal coughing, but a wheezing, rasping sort of coughing that you only hear when someone is gasping for breath. Even amid all the ear-shattering music the sound seemed to hold its own – I could even detect it with my earpiece in. I waited for a moment to see if it stopped, but it didn't – someone, somewhere, was in trouble.

I pulled out my earpiece and strained to hear where the sound of coughing was coming from. As I turned my head, the sound became more distinct and I followed it all the way to a dark alcove, near the edge of the dance floor. There, slumped in a gloomy corner, lay a middle-aged man fighting for breath. I knelt down and asked him what was wrong. With great difficulty, he pointed to his chest and murmured, "Tight." I'd seen the signs of heart trouble many times before and knew that he might be having a heart attack. The man was in severe pain and in no state to be moved, so I radioed for an ambulance and stayed by his side – overzealous clubbers were an unsafe stomping distance away.

The paramedics were quick to arrive and confirmed my suspicion that the man was having a heart attack. As they carried him out, one of the paramedics turned and said, "Thank God you got to him when you did. Any later could have been too late!"

Sound is a curious thing. Just as a soprano can still be heard above a full orchestra and chorus, so too can a quiet, but contrasting noise be heard above a much louder one. Learning to see with your ears is a precious skill to have. In the self-defence stakes, I'd put "earsight" higher up the scale than eyesight – with "earsight" your back is covered.

Chapter Four

COURTING DANGER – FOUR TRAPS

BEING UNCERTAIN

If you are uncertain about a decision, then it isn't worth going ahead with. Uncertain decisions always lead to uncertain actions, and if you are putting out uncertain actions, you will more than likely end up with something that you don't want. The stranger you have been chatting to for the last three hours wants to take you home, but you aren't sure what to do. While you take your time mulling it over, the stranger has made up your mind for you – very shaky ground to be on when it comes to your personal safety. Before you get roped into any situation that you might regret, ask yourself one thing: are you walking up the garden path of your own volition, or someone else's?

When you are uncertain about something it means that you are not in sync; it means that your body, mind, and spirit are not in agreement about some decision or other. As often as you can, stay in sync when making a decision. If even the tiniest part of you feels unsure about a choice, don't run with it – abort.

"I want them out and I want them out immediately!" boomed an exasperated head doorman in my earpiece one night. He'd tired of asking the only other female bouncer on duty to throw out two young women who were causing trouble, and was furious that the job still hadn't been done. Unluckily for me, the head doorman at that particular club considered me a sort of "bouncer's bouncer": any jobs that my colleagues couldn't get sorted would be dropped in my lap. Such was his frustration that the two young women were still inside the club, that he left his position at the front door, and followed me all the way to the dance floor to repeat his request. "Charly," he said, gasping for breath after having chased me up a couple

of flights of stairs, "the two young women I've asked Sandra to throw out are becoming a real problem. I've had so many complaints from the manager about them. Get them out asap will you?"

I caught up with my female colleague in the security room: she looked confused and thoroughly brassed off. "I'm sick of asking these two to leave," she sighed, pointing out the two young troublemakers with her radio antenna. "They're rude and keep hurling drinks at women in the ladies' loo."

It was clear that my colleague had bitten off far more than she could possibly chew. She'd dithered and been unsure about how to handle the situation, and the two young troublemakers were now taking advantage of the fact. Adamant that they weren't budging, they stood in the corner of the room like a couple of harpies and darted acid looks at her.

"We're not going, you cow!" carped one, sticking a perfectly manicured middle finger in the air.

"You can do what you want!" piped up the other one. "You're both f—g bitches! You'll never get us out!" With that, she plonked herself down on a sofa to make it quite clear that she wouldn't be leaving any time soon.

Now that I had the full measure of what I was up against, I walked straight over to both women and asked them to leave – they refused. I then outlined exactly what I was about to do: I'd give them to a count of three to decide whether they wanted to do things the easy way, or the difficult way. On the count of two, I moved in. I gently seized the first one by the arm, edged her through the door, up the stairs, and out onto the street faster than you could flick a feather duster. I raced back inside to deal with the second one. "It's time for —" Before I'd even finished my sentence, the young woman was already up and heading for the door. As I moved in to direct her to the stairs, she stiffened. "Don't – you – dare – touch me!" she shouted, dramatically lifting an indignant nose in the air. "I'll walk out on my own! Anything to get out of this dump!"

Being uncertain won't serve you. If you decide to give certainty a try, here's the recipe: use strategy, follow-through, and don't hesitate. Baking is not required as it is best served chilled.

PRIDE

A sensei once asked a whole class of students, "Which is more important: looking good, or winning?" Thirty replied that what mattered most was looking good. Only three of us answered winning. It seems to me that smacking an attacker in the face with a flip-flop – and surviving – is preferable to defending with a jumping, spinning side kick, and dying.

Indulging in pride will only make an argument worse. If a stranger abuses you verbally, and your pride is wounded, don't bite. Don't be provoked into replying with the same. Pride burns valuable energy, so don't fritter it away trying to get one up on your attacker. Things will almost certainly escalate if you do, and the one chance you had of escaping unharmed will elude you because you were too busy trying to make a point.

A domestic argument between a young couple erupted early one night in the lobby. It was an ugly scene: the verbal savagery being exchanged was enough to make even the sternest heart skip a beat. No sooner had the young pair run out of brutal things to say to each other, than the man decided to reinforce his point and went for the woman with his fist. Thankfully, the punch didn't land. While he was recoiling to strike again, the woman, without thinking, pulled a hairbrush out of her handbag and rammed it into the man's mouth. The force of it threw him back. He hit the wall behind him, crashed to the floor with a thud, and covered his face with his hands. While he was busy wallowing in pain and self-pity, the woman discreetly left, unhurt. I remember having nothing but admiration for her because she hadn't been too proud to rely solely on what worked – vanity hadn't got a look-in. When you let go of pride, you're the one still standing. And that's something to be proud of.

EGO

Absolutely nothing is personal. If a stranger disrespects you verbally then he becomes an open book, and you are privy to the state of his inner world. You only need a glimpse of a pitiful soul to realize that the abuse is about them – not you. Walk away from vitriol: the verbal bully is in a much worse state than you are.

The ego loves to hold onto pain. A lout insults you in a nightclub and you knee-jerk by wanting to pay him back – with interest. He has, after all, just laid some pretty nasty energy on you, and you want to send it back with torpedoes attached. I once had a very sinister interlude with a driver who thought I was driving in the wrong place, at the worst time. He pulled down his window and shouted every obscenity that he could think of. I pulled down my window and offered him a mint humbug. Theatrical displays of ego aren't really meant to be taken seriously. Treat them all with the lightness of being that they deserve, and concentrate instead on what really matters: your inner peace, your outward safety, and chocolate.

Having a large ego means you are self-important. Self-importance is very heavy; it takes real effort to carry it around everywhere. Why not give it the slip? Imagine life without all that extra load. Do yourself a favour and wave bye-bye to the Massive Ego Club. It isn't the best company in town anyway.

Bouncers would always come and go, and you never knew quite who you'd be working with next. I was running the doors one night when a very serious-looking Russian bouncer turned up for his first shift. He spoke very little English, so I stationed him just outside the front door with two of my crew, in the hope that they would break him in. My new recruit's body language was interesting: he parked himself in front of one of the metal barriers, and went to stone. Standing like a concrete block, the only part of him that moved were his eyes – I was heading a team of six bouncers and a monolith. I left him outside with my two colleagues to see how he got on, and disappeared inside to keep tabs on the rest of my team.

An hour later, I popped back out to have a word with my new Russian recruit. "Do you want to take a quick fifteen minutes?" I suggested. "Why don't you put your feet up for a bit?"

"Me, no need break," he replied, through gritted teeth. "Am strong. Not weak. Can stay all night long standing up." My serious Russian colleague

was obviously made of different stuff to the rest of us. I left him to his delusions and walked back inside.

I didn't leave it too long before sticking my head round the front door to see if he'd moved an inch from his spot. After three hours at the front door, my new recruit was still in the same place looking as stiff as a board; his face had crystallized into a menacing stare that fixed on any unfortunate passers-by – the man had granite for blood. It occurred to me that humour might be the best way to soften his hard outer shell – it was a tool I often used to relax my most self-important bouncers. "My friend," I asked, playfully, "how is it that you can stand still for so long? Are your feet nailed to the ground?" The serious Russian failed to see the funny side of my question. He threw me an icy glare and turned his back.

As humour hadn't succeeded in thawing him out, I fancied a change of scenery might – a spot of searching just inside the front door. Things only went from bad to worse: when a young prankster chucked my serious Russian colleague a cheeky one-liner while he was being frisked, he was grabbed, put in a tight headlock, and hurled straight over the metal barrier like a sack of potatoes. Even though the serious Russian spoke little English, he always assumed the worst. It worked for him. Making sure that every bout of pique got the better of him gave him all the licence he needed to throw his weight around.

I spent the rest of the night clearing up after my new Russian recruit. Wherever he went, trouble would always follow. A drug search on a polite young clubber was handled brutishly; a slightly tipsy young woman was frogmarched to the front door and thrown out as if she were a piece of trash. And so it went, with my Russian colleague never failing to choose the path of most resistance. The man was setting himself up for a monumental fall, though. Right after we closed, I took him into the security room. "I've just found out that you were caught on camera chucking that lad over the barrier. He will be prosecuting, of course." Once ego bites, it doesn't let go without a fight. It follows you around like a bad smell until either you fall, or everyone does.

CONTROL

It is futile to try and control anything. The only control you have is over yourself. A strange thing happens when you stop trying to control everything: you realize that there was never anything to control in the first place.

Real control isn't about surviving an attack: it is about preventing one. If you find yourself down a dark alley being attacked, don't fall into victim mode and ask, "Why me?" Ask yourself instead, "Why not me?" You took yourself to that spot; you walked there on your own two feet. The female warrior knows that in order to have any measure of control, she must have self-responsibility first. Ultimately, they are the same.

The way of real control is a paradox: in order to gain it, you have to let it go. This is a lesson that most people struggle with, and while a few are wise enough to learn it the easy way, most are predisposed to learn it the hard way. A friend of mine was no exception. She was in a violent relationship with a partner who had no qualms about beating her almost to death. What compounded her partner's sadistic outbursts was that she would try and get some sort of leverage over the situation. She would try, often aggressively, to put her partner off through words, ultimatums, or threats. None of it worked: she would either end up battered and broken, or find herself in Accident and Emergency.

One night while she was in the bedroom, her partner attacked. Before she'd even had time to defend herself with the hairbrush she was using, he picked her up by the scruff of the neck, threw her down on the bed, and got her in a stranglehold. My friend's instinct to resist immediately kicked in, which only made matters worse. The more she fought to break loose from her partner's hold, the more he tightened his grip.

My friend had been down this road before, and had always fought back. This time, death was so close she could feel it. With an overwhelming desire to live, she resorted to the only thing she had – surrender. She gave up the fight, went as limp as a rag doll, and played dead. Having nothing to fight against, her partner slowly began to release his grip. As he pulled away, my friend grabbed a thick buckled belt she had felt close to hand earlier on, and with as much willpower and courage as she could muster, whacked him in the face with it. As her partner lay semi-conscious on the floor, she called for help.

My friend took what she had learnt from this experience and used it to help her in every aspect of her life. And from then on, she became predisposed to do things the easy way.

The producers of a rave event got it badly wrong one night, when they sold too many tickets at one of Leicester Square's busiest nightclubs. The club's capacity was one and a half thousand, but nearly three thousand people turned up for the event. Security that night was no different to any other and as a result, we were dangerously understaffed. In no time, and through no fault of our own, the place was suddenly eight hundred over capacity. Before we'd had any time to halt the swelling tide of bodies all trying to squeeze in through the front doors, pandemonium broke out: women were getting trampled on, groups of men were laying into each other with knuckledusters – people were even jumping over the bars and stealing bottles of alcohol. A frantic head doorman called a code black over our radios, and every available bouncer raced inside in a vain attempt to establish some measure of order. Only two of us remained outside to stop a seven-hundred-strong angry mob from forcing its way in. Frenzied clubbers at the back of the crowd were now pushing the ones in front, and as we both fought to keep the mob from driving us back against the front doors, my colleague yelled, "Charly, I think we're going to lose this!"

"We already have!" I yelled back.

I had a decision to make right there and then: to either fight what was happening, or go with it. I quickly realized that I wasn't a strong enough swimmer to go against the tide, so I gave up the struggle and surrendered. A wall of bodies surged forward, pushed me back, and sent me flying backwards through the doorway. I now had less than a second to get out of the way before the desperate mob rushed in through the door. I threw myself to the side, grabbed two screaming women as I went, and stood, aghast, as the stampede thundered in.

There is some measure of irony to this story: while we'd been opening up earlier on, I'd mentioned to a colleague that thousands might turn up – we'd heard a rumour to that effect. My fellow bouncer didn't seem fazed. "Huge crowds? We'll get it sorted! We'll just give 'em some of that!" he said, waving an aggressive fist in the air. "Anyway, babe," he continued, winking at me as if he knew something that the world and God didn't, "I've 'ad plenty of crowds at the doors before – piece of p—s!"

The man had taken leave of his senses. As far as he was concerned, fifteen "iron-pumping" bouncers were more than enough to keep thousands of rebellious clubbers in line. "A cinch!" he added, strutting around like an overexcited silverback.

I suppose pushing weights five nights a week down at the local gym made my colleague invincible. I, however, was not. After we'd finally closed, and after what must have been one of the darkest hours of my career as a bouncer, I'd had enough and was ready for home. I passed my invincible colleague as I was leaving: he was now sitting at the bar holding a badly fractured wrist – a far cry from the overexcited silverback that he'd been only hours before. He avoided my gaze as I patted him on the back. "Impressive crowd control, mate," I said, taking advantage of the fact that he only had one hand left to strike with. "Those muscles of yours served you well."

Chapter Five

YOUR BODY, YOUR GUARDIAN

BODY INTELLIGENCE

You have two intelligences: mind intelligence, and body intelligence. When it comes to your personal safety, you really only have one intelligence worth trusting: body intelligence. Your mind can trip you up when it comes to identifying either potential or actual danger, and while the body understands the now of things, the mind wastes precious time worrying about yesterday and tomorrow. When you are in possible danger, you usually don't have much time to waste on thinking, but when danger strikes, you have none – thinking costs.

You will be so much safer if you trust what your body's intelligence is telling you. I once walked out of a dojo halfway through a class. I told my sensei that I didn't want to take another grading as I was happy with the blue belt I already had. I was also quite content with the ten defence techniques I had, thank you very much. He was outraged, and tried to insult me into seeing things his way. I was "strong, but stupid", and was "slow to pick up". He added that I needed to get to black belt level so that I would have hundreds of techniques under my belt – so to speak. I made my apologies and headed for the door. I knew then, as I do now, that had I had hundreds of techniques under my belt, I would have got badly hurt while trying to decide which one of them to use. My mind would have been in the driving seat, rather than my body.

It doesn't pay to let your mind override what intelligence comes to you from your body. Your body has a sophisticated warning system in place that can be relied on to keep you out of harm's way. When it sets alarm bells ringing, make sure you are tuning in.

Not listening to my body's warning system one night cost me dearly. I was running the doors at one of London's most notorious nightclubs – bouncers at the venue were often referred to as "minced beef" – and it was up to me to train a new recruit. I was stationed at the front door with my inexperienced colleague introducing him to a few important house rules

when a young man, who I'd barred only weeks before for buying and using drugs while inside the nightclub, turned up demanding to be let in. Visibly shaking from the lack of a fix, the young drug addict quickly checked himself, thought better of trying to bully his way in and, feigning politeness, asked to be allowed in. While he'd always had a wild stare, that night there was madness in his eyes. He stood in the doorway devouring the view of goings-on inside. The fix he so badly needed was a skip and a jump away; it was so close he could almost touch it, but for me standing in his way.

I refused the young drug addict entry in the same mild-mannered way I always had, and while part of me sensed that he hadn't come to plead but to menace, another part of me foolishly allowed him to hover near the front door. I turned around to continue showing my new recruit the ropes, when I overheard the young drug addict muttering obscenities at me under his breath – he'd sunk to a new low. I didn't take any of this seriously. I felt sure he would eventually talk himself out. This was one of the poorest judgement calls I was ever to make. With a wail loud enough to wake the dead, the young drug addict charged towards me, spread open his palm an inch from my face, and told me I'd be feeling the hard side of it if I didn't let him in. All this should have been proof enough that I was now in the presence of a raging lunatic. There is a paper-thin line, though, between procrastination and denial, and that night I strayed too far into both. And my body knew it: a light-headedness, and a spring in my step equal to any gazelle's were the same clarion calls as ever to defensive action. But I drowned out my body's knowing, swept all danger under the carpet, and carried on regardless.

Things were cranking up a gear at the front door. The long queue of bolshie youngsters all needing to be searched was now a quarter of a mile long, and growing. I waved over a young woman and asked her to open her bag, but before I'd even started searching her, the young drug addict pushed in front and ordered me to frisk him first. As if he was done talking, he stood in the doorway fixing me with sunken eyes and a maniacal grin. I told him to back away from the door, and stay there. When he did nothing, I got hold of him and moved him there myself. Everything in me was telling me to get help and have the man removed, but I didn't. I buried my head in the sand, ignored my body's inner promptings, and continued showing my new recruit how to deal with a drunken man who was now refusing to cooperate. I was halfway through helping him out, when suddenly, from my left, the incensed drug addict swung for my face. The punch landed –

hard. These days, whenever my body sends me postcards, I read them.

GUT FEELING

If you find yourself alone on a street and sense that you are being followed, then you probably are. Even if you feel you have misjudged the situation, immediately cross over to the other side of the street – create as much distance as you can. All gut feeling is worthy of being taken seriously. If any defensive action you take *feels* right, then it is.

Stop for a moment to consider whether you are making decisions because of something you think you *should* do, or because of something you truly *want* to do. The first line of decision making has been enforced from without; the second is motivated from within – one is from outside, the other is from inside. A gut decision is always a superior one because it means you are acting from within – the fire that you feel in your belly confirms that you are coming from your own truth. Trusting your gut is a way to steer a free course through life, and true.

Having the courage to rely on my gut instinct got me out of no end of trouble on the doors. Every time I felt my solar plexus or belly start to bubble and churn like an engine room on an ocean liner, that would be my cue to either disappear, or prepare to defend. I kept this in mind one night when I turned up for my first shift at a new nightclub in London. I was booked there for the whole weekend – ironically, I didn't make it to the second night. As soon as I walked in, something about the place just made me uneasy. A cold dampness blew over me like a foul wind – even the air smelled of doom.

Living up to my reputation as a true pro, I tucked my radio into my belt, fitted my earpiece in place, and headed for my station at the bar. As I walked, I scanned as much of the area as I could and while everything still appeared to be ticking over as it should, I knew something wasn't right. The butterfly belly I'd had on entering was now doing a Highland jig in my gut: my belly was obviously seeing something my eyes couldn't.

As we began showing people out at the end of the night, I was more unsettled than ever and decided to act on that feeling. Before leaving, I made my apologies to the head doorman and told him that I wouldn't be back. He shrugged his shoulders, chucked me a wry smile, and offered me a lukewarm "so long".

A week later, I opened a local newspaper to read that the very same nightclub had been closed down: a fire had swept through the place the night after I'd left. No one was killed, but quite a few people were badly injured, including some of the doormen.

Chapter Six

YOUR WORD AS YOUR SHIELD

THE POWER OF WORDS

Never underestimate the power of your words. Your words, and how you use them, can often influence whether a street thug will attack or not. At the verbal stage of any confrontation, try doing the opposite of what you might usually do. This will make you unpredictable, and it will also confuse your average attacker. When you start speaking don't speed up, but instead slow down. Make sure your words are deliberate, and steady. Become very present as you talk – your average attacker won't be expecting this. He will be expecting you to panic. Maintaining your balance in the face of danger, even with your words, is a forceful defence.

You need every bit of energy to keep safe when you are out and about. The words you choose, and how you say them, can either bring it to you, or take it away. Clear and inoffensive language brings you energy. When you resist the temptation of shouting all manner of verbal nasties at people, you keep your life force – you stay centred and intact. Aggressive, hostile words, on the other hand, rob you of energy. It isn't hard to see why: it takes a lot out of you when you hurl abuse at someone. When you verbally batter an opponent you work terribly hard, and you end up not only losing precious calories, but your power to boot.

So be mindful of what you say and how you say it. If you feel yourself starting to flare up when someone gives you a verbal lashing, just remember that when you indulge in any mud-slinging, you lose control. Without that, you are less likely to follow through with an appropriate defence. When you verbally disrespect others, it weakens you. It brings you closer to the firing line.

"I don't think this club is the right place for you. I know you really don't

want to come in here. Please leave." These were the words I firmly, but quietly, repeated over and over again to an intruder one night. I was running the doors at a small club in west London, and had been opening up. My back hadn't been turned a few seconds when a stranger silently crept in. The tall, heavyset intruder stood in the lobby and proceeded to quiz me about the venue. He made no eye contact while I answered his questions, but just scanned the place as if making quite sure I was alone. When he was satisfied that I was, he cut his interrogation dead, spun around, and with hungry eyes stared at me, transfixed. It wasn't my demeanour or character that was being studied: it was my soul. With empty, cold eyes that hardly blinked, the intruder's stare cut through to a raw, fragile place. He settled in that fragility and seemed to breathe it in, as if feeding off it. But fragility wasn't to be his only food: nourishment would be had from any opportunity to abuse and terrify. A blood rush, and a heightened state of alertness hit as I realized that the intruder hadn't come to party: he'd come to do the devil's work.

The shock had me feeling so light that I felt as if I were floating three feet in the air. I was so punch-drunk with dread of what might be, that I only just found the wherewithal to ask the intruder to leave a second time. "As I've already said, I don't think this club is the right place for you. I can tell you really don't want to come in here. Leave – please." The intruder cracked a soulless smile, crossed his arms, and pitched camp – this reptile from the underworld had no intention of going anywhere. He'd scurried in through the door to see what plaything he could find and use to spread mayhem. His devilish assignment was only beginning.

The intruder was a cat playing with a mouse, and was in no hurry to carry out what he'd been sent to do. He closed his eyes, inhaled the exquisite tension of the moment, and feasted – a dramatic pause to amplify the unholy assault that was to follow. When he was ready, the intruder snapped himself to attention, looked at me, stalk-eyed, and poured out a torrent of verbal abuse that I'd never come across in my years as a bouncer – an onslaught that continued unabated for fifteen minutes. Each insult was punctuated with enough venom to demolish the hardiest of spirits. This servant of Hades was wielding his words like a sickle to torture and break my will. I felt alone and utterly defenceless. I was trapped in some giant bell jar with a monstrous entity on a mission to destroy me. I couldn't be seen or heard. I was dead to the world.

The extraordinary can come out of a seemingly hopeless situation. Something occurred to me that ran completely contrary to what was *actually happening. It struck me that maybe I wasn't alone. Perhaps there was some hidden ally that I could call on to help me now. I dug deep to find the sort of courage that stops you from writing scripts and assuming the worst. Refusing to be influenced by the fact that I had nothing to defend myself with – I didn't have so much as a stool or a chair to hand as the entrance was bare – I put all doubt to one side and contemplated the absurd. I would trust in the integrity and power of the only thing that I had – words.*

I faced the intruder square on, and spoke. As he vented his rage, I continued my steady patter. With every negative from him, came a positive from me. Every evil he spewed was met with a determined, but courteous reply, and neutralized. And in direct proportion to his growing hostility, my words became measured, slow, and solid. In the face of a fifteen minute blast of the darkest energy, I'd countered each of the intruder's verbal strikes using the power of my words as a shield.

As if Hades himself was instructing him from the deep, the intruder froze. He lifted his nose as if checking to see which way the wind was blowing, turned on his heels, and headed for the door. Exasperated that I'd stoically stood my ground, he crawled out into the night, with his tail between his legs.

SPEAKING FROM YOUR BODY

Street predators attack vulnerable women because they can easily overpower them. A street predator can tell how vulnerable you are by how you use your voice. If you aren't speaking from your body – from your power base – he will know it because you will be talking from the neck up. Women who speak from the neck up often have squeaky and breathy voices; their words only resonate in their throat and mouth. If you don't want to appear vulnerable to an attacker, use your whole body to speak. Many physical attacks on women begin with a conversation and if you are speaking from your body at this point, things are far less likely to get physical.

It is only possible to speak from your body when your body, mind, and spirit are all operating as a single unit. If those three parts are not working in tandem, then you are split. Think about it: if your words are saying one thing, but your feelings and body language are saying another, then you are multitasking.

It isn't difficult to tell when you are speaking from your body. When the gap almost closes between what you are thinking and feeling, and what is coming out of your mouth, you are using your body to speak. When the mind gets involved in that process, your body's integrity is interrupted, and unity goes out of the window.

When you use your whole body to speak, you are left with a lot more energy to play with – multitasking is hard work. All that extra va-va-voom can be liberating: suddenly, you have turbocharged reserves of power at your fingertips. You have been driving a car around all this time thinking it was a Fiat Panda, when in fact, what you really have is a Ferrari.

So hold it all together. Ensure that your body, mind, and spirit are all singing from the same hymn book. And keep any multitasking strictly for the kitchen.

To see how it feels physically to speak from your body, place your fingers on your solar plexus, just beneath your sternum. Let out a few ha-has and feel the action that follows there – that is your diaphragm at work. Now there is something that supports the diaphragm: your lower belly. Put your fingers there, just above your pubic bone, and let out a few more ha-has – that is the womb area of your belly. You will feel the muscles there pop in and out as they move in unison with your diaphragm. Your lower belly supports all the upper parts when you produce any sound. When you are speaking from there, you are speaking from your centre – a woman's place of power lies in her womb. When you connect with that place, you will know what speaking from your body is all about. Animals do it automatically – ever wondered how a small bird can make so much noise?

We were only minutes away from closing one night, and things at the front door were slowly beginning to wind down. I often liked to amble up to the front door for a moment of stillness before leaving. I'd soak up the tranquillity of the atmosphere outside, and switch back into the calm mood that I'd arrived in.

I happened to be standing outside a few feet away from the entrance, when my reverie was cut short by the strident voices of two female colleagues trying to stop an intoxicated clubber from walking back inside. He'd keep having a last go at creeping back in and was fast becoming a pest. "Stay away from the door. One more time and you're barred," said one of the two female bouncers nonchalantly, with her back turned. She was busy having a chinwag with one of the regulars and didn't give the matter a second thought. The man took no notice and continued edging towards the front door. "Go home. You're drunk. Way past your bedtime," mumbled the other. She'd been a bouncer for some months but now hated it. With her heart no longer in the job, she was too bored to even care whether the drunken man sneaked his way back inside or not.

The man was now within five paces of the door and, not surprisingly, hadn't been deterred a jot. "Charly, can you please get this git to back away from the door? He just won't listen," pleaded one of my colleagues. "If the head doorman catches him back inside, we'll be in the soup!" she added, turning away to enjoy some more gossip from the regular.

With a gentle, but deliberate step, I walked up to within a foot of the man and faced him. "My friend, it's time for you to go home. We both know where you belong, and it's not here. Step away from the door, please."

Every inch of me was speaking these words. I was using my entire body as a platform to deliver them. It was then that I realized something incredible: my words weren't merely sounds, they were things – it was as if they were solid. The man I was speaking to reacted as if they had been. Without me even touching him, he suddenly staggered backwards, and reached behind for a metal barrier that wasn't there. He lost his footing, slipped on the curb, and landed on his backside. Cursing all the while, he clambered to his feet, paused for a moment to decide whether or not to fight for his lost pride, then wisely chose to head for the nearest tube station and return home. The bewilderment on the man's face as he took a tumble was something I'll never forget. Out of the two of us, I think I was the more shocked.

WORD FOR WORD

An attacker often uses words to groom and single out a potential victim. The words he chooses, and the way they are spoken, is significant – as is the quantity of them. An endless stream of questions or seemingly harmless banter is a deliberate ploy to disempower you. When you are at a bar and a man asks you if you would like a drink, make sure he gives you time to answer. If he is talking over you as you tell him you don't want one, just match him word for word. Repeat no again and again – nothing else, just *no*. No need to shout or get angry. Just firmly say no over and over as if you are a record that has got stuck. You are then pushing out a continuous drone of chatter to mirror his; you are creating a fence with words. If a man isn't able to dominate you with words, he is less likely to try and dominate you in any other way.

No, I wasn't going to let an underager into the bar. Local councils don't take kindly to underage drinkers, and will think nothing of closing down a bar if they are found drinking in these places on a regular basis. The lad I'd refused entry to loitered near the entrance for an age. He'd outstayed his welcome and was becoming tiresome, not in an angry or violent way, but in a whining, moaning sort of way that only comes from the mouths of spoilt babes. He parked himself near my side of the front door in order to harass me, and proceeded to bombard me with one vacuous question after another. In order to shut the teenybopper up, I ignored all his questions. This, however, was only adding petrol to the fire.

"Tell me why you won't let me in!" he ranted, patting down his kiss curl to make himself look a few years older. "Tell me what gives you the right to discriminate against young people!"

"No identification, no entry. That is the law," I calmly reminded him.

"I'm a regular here!" he shrieked, stamping a pristine sneaker up and down. "I know the manager! Go and get him! He knows how old I am! Everyone here knows I'm over eighteen! It's – not – fair!"

Briefly, he went quiet. The cogs of his underage mind slowly started to turn as it dawned on him that no tantrum, however spectacular, would sway me into letting him in. It was then that he got nasty. He slowly looked me up and down, and smirked as if he'd found a weakness to play on. "You're new here, aren't you?"

That was it. The brat had given me a headache, and it was high time he had a taste of his own medicine. In order to take the wind out of his sails, I subjected him to an endless stream of nos. I repeated no to every word that came out of the teenybopper's mouth. While he was talking, I was saying no. When he wasn't talking, I continued saying no. When he occasionally stopped for breath, all he could hear was me saying no. About fifty nos later, the boy's attention slackened. Mid-question, he got bored, singled out someone else to give an earbashing to, and wandered off.

PROJECTING SPEECH

When people take themselves seriously, they project their words. When they project their words, they are taken seriously. Begin by taking yourself seriously if you want others to. As soon as you do, you will be amazed at how easy it is to command attention. Projecting your words is the difference between keeping them to yourself, and allowing them to travel outwards to the world. Unconsciously, people who mumble don't want to share what they are saying. This is why most people aren't too bothered if they don't hear something that has been mumbled. They know that if a person mumbles, they aren't serious about being heard.

People who project what they are saying are quite the opposite: they want people to listen – and people will. Often, they won't know why they are listening, but they will be drawn to you anyway. This is because when you project as you speak, your words hold more life force – it is that energy that people are attracted to. It is that energy that also acts as a defence against potential attack. Street predators can tell how much life force you have by whether you verbally project or not. If they hear you project as you speak, they will almost certainly leave you alone. All street thugs are cowards, and if they hear you project verbally, many of them will see you as having far more life force than they are prepared to take on.

The best way to project your words is to make sure they are soft, slow, and have weight. Putting weight into your words might not come naturally. As you speak, imagine them as having dumb-bells attached to them. That will slow things down a tad, and will give you added impetus. Soft, slow, and heavy words will give a potential attacker three clear messages: softness tells him you are powerful enough not to be spooked, slowness tells him you will not be rushed, and verbal gravitas tells him you mean business. If I were a street thug, I wouldn't mess with that.

Projecting your words is a bit like aiming an arrow at a target. Become an archer with your words, and always make sure they land.

A call on my radio had me running to the security office: two colleagues needed assistance with a drug search. After catching a young man buying cocaine inside the club, they'd been pressing him for twenty minutes, without success, to empty his pockets.

These two particular colleagues were known to have the shortest tempers on the team: it was vital that I got there before they resorted to their usual bully boy methods for dealing with troublemakers. When I arrived, I was almost relieved to find that it was stalemate. The young clubber, who thought of himself as a bit of a wide boy, knew that he was on camera and couldn't be forced to do anything. He stood in the middle of the room texting on his mobile phone, and refused to cooperate. I asked my two colleagues to leave the young man with me. I wanted to try another tactic and wear down the young know-all – if I could.

As the door closed, I warmly invited the young man, who was still punching out a message on his mobile, to take a seat. With his eyes glued to his phone, he reached behind, fumbled around for a chair, and plonked himself down. I perched myself on a table next to him, and said nothing. I wanted silence in the room so that when I spoke, my voice would cut through it like a knife. I waited. Then, hoping that my words alone would be enough to soften the young man's guard, I slowly and quietly asked him to empty his pockets. While he didn't agree to this, neither did he refuse. I repeated my request a second time, and slowed down my words even more by giving them as much weight, and purpose, as I could. As if a spell had been broken, the young know-all's texting stopped. Still looking down at his mobile, he swayed back and forth like a petulant teenager waiting to see what punishment an angry parent would be dishing out.

My words, evidently, were having an effect. Like the steady motion of water over unforgiving rock, they were eroding the young man's hard outer crust. With words that held all the gentleness and intensity of the ages, I asked the young man a third time to empty his pockets. It was so quiet in the room that I could hear the faint sizzling of the light bulb filament above, as it swung to and fro. The young man's rocking petered out, he settled, and instead of trying to avoid my gaze, he now looked up at me for the first time. As he did, I said, "Please empty your pockets for me.

Do this now and we can —" Before I'd finished my sentence, the young know-all had emptied his pockets, and put what shouldn't have been in them on the table.

Chapter Seven

THE SOFTENING BEGINS

BEING PRESENT

You cannot protect yourself if you are not taking in what is happening around you. Being fully present enables you to do this. When you are fully present, you are giving whatever you are doing your complete attention. This is the state you need to be in when you are defending against an attack. If an attacker strikes, you need the presence of mind to concentrate not on what he *might* do, but on what he *is* doing. Being fully present gives you the moment. That is where you must meet your attacker, if you are to survive.

To connect fully to the present, do a simple exercise: on a warm, sunny day go outside in nature and sit yourself down somewhere quiet, where you won't be disturbed. When the wind picks up, see if you can feel it gently brushing your cheek. Open to the wind's soft touch on your skin. You will then understand that being present is not about your body mass acting on space: it is space exerting itself on you. When you are able to experience this, you will know how to be present.

Very quickly, but silently, a young man crept in through the door. His dress code was shabby and anyway we were closing, so I asked him to leave. He just stood not uttering a word, and stared. While he made no attempt to move forward, he was clearly standing his ground. "Do you speak English?" I asked. He nodded yes.
Not so much as a quiver of a lip came from the gaunt face that was fixing me. Could he be on drugs? Was he carrying a knife? Would he attack? The intensity of the moment shut out everything but my fear, and while my head was telling me not to face all this alone, another part of me kept me

planted to the spot. In all my years on the doors, this was the most terrified I'd ever been. I was scared to my bones. I was also losing my nerve.

The mute stranger was still ominously scrutinizing me from only ten feet away. It crossed my mind that his arrival was personal: perhaps a grudge that needed sorting had brought him to my door. I pressed myself to make a decision.

"For God's sake, woman, get a grip. Either sling him out, or face whatever comes."

I stayed put. Not even a dry mouth and plasticine legs that were about to give way could induce me to budge. I was locked in a stand-off and mirroring the stranger stare for stare – I couldn't have torn myself away even if I'd wanted to. This impasse, as it turned out, was a gift: the weight of fear became so great that I just couldn't hold it any longer. As fear began to leave, courage, and an uncompromising gall, took its place. All dread, fear of what might be, and worry, simply vanished. In an instant, blinding flash of pure presence, everything collapsed – except the moment. One moment had stretched so far into infinity that it took me to a profound state of grace. Nothing mattered anymore. I didn't even care if help arrived or not.

I was still standing eyeball to eyeball with the stranger, only it wasn't fear that now fuelled my stare, but faith. The stranger, motionless as a waxwork dummy, watched as I watched him. The two of us, actors in some cosmic drama, were performing outside of time and all human concern. Our invisible exchange wasn't bound by time or space, but by spirit. In order to test the strength of the stranger's spirit pitched against mine, I ordered him to leave a second time. The stranger wasn't done: his higher purpose was almost fulfilled, but not quite. He shook his head and remained rooted to the floor.

Like a warrior who has nothing more to lose, I continued holding my space. I'd travelled through fear to the other side, and had settled utterly within the present. My surrender must have shown because without warning, the intruder broke his stare. As if some Godly arbitrator had shattered our window of timelessness, he stiffened, straightened his back, and tilted his head as if checking me out one last time for any chinks in my armour. Convinced that my focus had remained solid, and that my resolve to stay purely in the moment hadn't worn down, his fierce expression softened. With a satisfied smirk, my unexpected visitor gestured a flamboyant salute, bowed respectfully, and left as silently as he'd arrived.

THE ADVANTAGE OF DEFENCE OVER ATTACK

If a person tries to attack you, they pay dearly for the privilege for they have fixed their energy in one place. As the defender, you are free to move anywhere you choose.

It is as easy as pie to unbalance someone who is moving at the speed of an express train. It is all about inertia. The faster someone moves, the more energy and time they need to slam on the breaks. An attacker races towards you: all you need to do to make him go flying is to shift to the side, and shove him from there as he rushes past. It takes far less effort than you imagine to redirect him this way. I once tried this while training in a dojo. A huge lump of a lad came hurtling towards me as we practised some grappling drills. He was surprisingly light on his feet, and moved in fast to grab my jacket and throw me down on the mat. As he continued on his forward trajectory, I switched to a circular one. Just before he reached me, I moved around to the side of him and pushed the side of his knee with the flat of my foot. That was enough to send him off at a tangent. He landed face down in a male student's lap on the other side of the mat.

If an attacker approaches at lightning speed, don't be fooled into thinking that he has more power than you. If you have balance over speed, then *you* have the edge.

When a street thug attacks, he generates a huge amount of energy trying to annihilate you. This can be a great advantage because as the defender, you have added energy to draw from – he has enough for the both of you. Think of it as surfing: you use the ocean's power to crest the top of each wave as it arrives. A street thug grabs you by the wrist, and forcefully pulls you towards him – don't resist. Allow yourself to be flung and, using the energy of his pull as momentum, elbow him in the face with your free arm as you close in. Nabbing an attacker's energy is smart: with the extra boost, you are more likely to trot out a defence that will count. Never feel guilty about using some of your attacker's energy – he is coming after yours!

The phone rang just before I left for work. The head doorman at a club I was working at had an emergency to deal with and would be an hour late – could I hold the front door till he arrived? Without hesitation, I said yes. On my way to the central London club I promised myself that I'd be extra vigilant: holding the front door was dangerous enough under normal circumstances, but manning it on my own, even for an hour, was risky.

As soon as I arrived I set up outside. I didn't want any hoodlums kicking up a storm as they entered the place – at least not until the head doorman arrived. Using some metal barriers, I herded a group of noisy clubbers into a neat queue that skirted the outside of the club, took a deep breath, and swung open the front door for the melee to pile in. The door hadn't been open ten minutes when a young toothless wonder, with more swagger than he knew what to do with, tried to barge in without being searched. Spurred on by the fact that there was no head doorman in sight, and only a woman to stop him reaching the dance floor, he decided to take advantage of what he saw as an easy target. As soon as my back was turned, the young toothless wonder took a running jump and hurled himself through a narrow gap in the doorway behind me.

Little did he know that I'd dealt with the antics of young pups before – and on my own. As he shot through the door, I caught the back of his coat collar, and with a quick, light tug from behind, pulled him off balance. The young toothless wonder did a clumsy pirouette, and spun like a top all the way back out. There were many magical moments on the doors, but this ranked as one of the most priceless because until that moment, I'd never physically achieved so much, using so little.

The bewildered youngster collected himself, dusted himself down, and shook with rage. The disgrace of having been thrown out bodily – and by a woman – was too much. I wondered if he'd try to even things up with a punch. A second later, with his arm pointing forward to strike, he came for me. I saw the punch coming, moved an inch to the side, and watched him fly past, straight into the glass front door behind me. He hit the door with an almighty crack, and stood blaming all the world but himself for his demise. "Look what you've done to me you f—g bitch!" he yelped. "My face is cut and my wrist is probably f—g broken!"

"Don't credit me with all that," I replied. "You did all the hard work. I just helped you along a little."

BAGGING HEAVINESS

Attackers use force to disempower you. A lot of effort and calories are spent while they do this. It is tempting to follow suit – try not to. Just rely on your feminine heritage, and apply softness to respond. Losing any of your lightness will not serve you. A thought is weightless; a punch is heavy. You can think faster than your attacker can strike. There is safety in a feather-light touch.

While it is usually considered an insult to tell someone that they are communing with the fairies, I wouldn't dismiss the expression in a hurry. The wonderful thing about fairyland is that fairies get to fly off. Feminine energy is like that: as nimble as it comes. From the safety point of view, it doesn't get better than that.

Two rotund doormen were making extremely heavy work of removing a nine stone weakling from an entrance staircase one night. The man in question was somewhat worse for wear, and my two colleagues decided that he'd had quite enough – a featherweight's measure of alcohol, no doubt – and it was high time he left. The skinny clubber was having none of it. Shouting his refusal to move an inch, his hands latched onto the banister as if his life depended on it. My colleagues, who were a rather portly, well fed couple, resorted to drastic measures: one would take hold of the man's left leg, and the other would do the same on the other side. With a weight differential of at least twenty stone in their favour, they'd have him out in a jiffy.

Ten minutes later, my two fellow bouncers were still heaving and pouring sweat over a job that should have taken a fraction of the time to put right. I happened, by chance, to be walking nearby during all this carry-on, and caught sight of my two colleagues making a meal of it all. Another case of brawn triumphing over brain, I feared – should I offer some assistance? I strolled down the staircase to see what I could do. My two chubby colleagues were now going puce with the strain of trying to tear the featherweight away from the banister. In a bizarre twist of fate, the defiant thinnifer's resolve was growing. Now clinging on by his fingers, he

*squealed like a banshee with every tug, and prayed for divine intervention
with every pull. The waif's pleas for mercy were so piercing, that even
passers-by outside stopped and ogled through the glass front doors to
witness, what they thought, was a murder being committed. In order to
prevent my eardrums, and the two glass front doors, from shattering, I
approached my two colleagues and offered them an alternative to using
force. The heavy-handed approach to door supervision hadn't worked,
after all, and the whole matter needed immediate closure. I gently got hold
of one of the clubber's thumbs to pull it back into a lock, but before I'd
applied any real pressure, he released his grip, and as fast as a shot from
a gun, all three careered out through the door and landed in a messy heap
outside. From the pavement, a pained, muffled voice cried out for help.
The featherweight had ended up in between the two heavyweights, and got
stuck. There he was, a thin layer of beef, sandwiched between two fat,
warm, bouncy rolls.*

NO-FORCE SOLUTIONS

When people rely only on force, they limit their range of defences. Try
something that has worked for me for many years: use soft on hard, and hard on
soft. Let me explain: you can knock an attacker unconscious with surprisingly
little force. A fast, deft, concentrated palm or elbow strike to the chin is enough
to get the job done. On the other hand, a hard finger jab to someone's eyeball is
all you need to shift the balance of power considerably in your favour. This is
distribution of force at its best. It is what I call "powder puff" self-defence – my
favourite.

It used to take me ages to undo a knotted shoelace. I would try and get a knot
untangled by being rude and obnoxious to it. Shoelaces don't take kindly to
being insulted, so one day I tried a different approach. I lovingly, softly, and
caringly, untangled a knot. My shoelaces were not offended, and I got the job
done in half the time.

One of the most colourful nightspots I worked at was an enormous venue in a part of London called Embankment. Serial clubbers of every description would come from far and wide to drink at that particular watering hole. I liked the place because whether you were straight, gay, or transgender, you'd always be made to feel at home – you were accepted no matter what. Big, hairy truck drivers with pink petticoat dresses on and long blond wigs, would totter in on eight inch heels; butch women with stares that would make even the strongest of the security team quake, would walk in as if they owned the place. There was a lot of everything at that nightclub – including trouble.

The venue was so big that it even had a huge cafe. One night, while ordering a coffee during my break, I happened to notice a man sitting a few feet away, hurling abuse at everyone and flicking cigarette butts at them as they walked by – no one was safe. I hadn't been the first to notice him either. "Charly! Get rid of the fat t—r in the coffee shop! 'E's been causing trouble for ages!" barked the club manager in my earpiece. He'd already asked several of my colleagues to remove the troublemaker and was seething that the job still hadn't been done. "Is he the f—g incredible bulk or what?" he yelled. "Get the fat git out now!"

Why my colleagues hadn't removed the man was a complete mystery, but all that mattered now was to focus on the job in hand, and try to keep a furious club manager sweet. "Don't worry," I assured him, "I'll get him out."

Assured I wasn't. If my colleagues hadn't managed to throw out the troublemaker, what chance would I have? I suspended my doubt, put down my coffee, and walked straight towards the troublemaker, who was now making crude gestures at a pale, shy young man sitting at the next table. As soon as the bully saw me coming, he sunk his corpulent frame even deeper into his chair, grabbed his panama, and hid underneath it in the hope of becoming invisible. The man was in no mood to be ousted from his seat.

Nevertheless, I gave him the benefit of the doubt, and politely asked him to leave. "The manager has asked me to escort you to the door. I would be grateful if you would come with me, please." A predictable two-fingered salute followed. While I was twiddling my thumbs wondering what to do next, I found myself staring at the man's mobile phone – he'd left one of the fanciest I'd ever seen on the table in front of him. It was so fancy, that I picked it up and played with it all the way to the front door and beyond. With surprisingly little effort, the belligerent heavyweight hauled himself up, and followed me there, screaming for his mobile phone all the way.

BEING SILENT

If you are having a verbal fight with someone, the one thing that will most often take it to the next level – a physical confrontation – is words. If a stranger is planning an attack, he must close the gap between you and will often use words to do this. The words are a bridge: one minute the stranger you are talking to is six feet away, and the next, you find yourself within inches of him.

Words are the fuel that brings a potential attacker close enough to hurt you physically. It is wise to keep silent if someone you don't know tries to strike up a conversation with you in a public place. If he is over there, and you are over here, keep it that way. When you kill talk, you also kill danger.

Silent power is a major player in your bag of personal safety tricks. Walking in silence is an intelligent way to nip danger in the bud, because endless chatter drowns out a lot of ambient sounds that could alert you to danger. You always need to be able to hear the footsteps of others when you are out alone, late at night.

Choosing to be silent, rather than talking non-stop, also makes you appear mysterious and contained; you project inner strength when you do this. Have you ever noticed how much more of an impact people make when they don't gush verbally?

Being silent also means that you will be more likely to pass unnoticed under the street attacker's nose, because he is trying to single out a chatterbox – someone he can creep up on, unawares.

To keep us occupied on quiet nights, my colleagues and I used to exchange opinions and stories about our skills as martial artists. In my innocence, I used to imagine that sharing dojo banter with them would make me one of the team – I couldn't have been more wrong. Whenever trouble erupted, I was nearly always the last to know. Every door supervisor except me would be alerted, and I'd be landed with front door duty while my

colleagues rushed inside to do all the serious bouncing. The fact that I had three black belts to my name, and legs strong enough to push well over two hundred kilogrammes on the leg press, didn't sway their preconceived ideas any. I wasn't to be included when physical violence broke out, and that was that. I finally cottoned on and gave up spilling the beans about what I was capable of. I was tired of trying to prove that I could cut the mustard with the toughest of them.

One night on my first shift at a new club, I decided to play things differently and keep all my "savoir faire" to myself. I played dumb. Not offering information about myself freely, however, made my colleagues try all the more to get me to open up. Bouncers are often a competitive lot, and are keen to know what their colleagues are made of on the self-defence front. As I stood at the front door guarding the entrance with one of my new team, he threw so many personal questions at me that I felt dizzy. "Charly," he inquired, pushing his head forward like a cockerel in a henhouse, "you 'ad any martial arts training, babe?"

I pretended I didn't know what he meant. "No, I haven't," I replied. "I am familiar with marital arts, though." Satisfied that I knew nothing on the subject, he strolled back inside, leaving me in peace to guard the front door.

Moments later, a man walked in with a bottle of wine sticking out of his pocket. I politely asked him to hand me the bottle before going inside, but not only did he refuse, he took a swipe at me with it. Just before the bottle came crashing down on my head, I jumped behind him, grabbed the bottle, and with a slight downward tug, pulled him off balance. The man staggered backwards, tripped over his own feet, and released the bottle as he fell.

My plan to keep my martial arts knowledge under wraps didn't last long after that. A colleague, who'd been rushing in to help, had witnessed me single-handedly disarming my attacker, and in no time, my fortuitous brush with danger was on every bouncer's lips. It made quite an impact, though. After an entire night of front door duty – colleagues had spread the word that I was now to be called the standing stone of the south-east – the head doorman burst through the inner doors, and like a commander rallying his finest troops, yelled, "Charly! Get inside! There's half a dozen blokes in there who think there's a war on! I need you on the dance floor!"

That night I made a much bigger splash keeping quiet about what I knew. And from then on, I was usually the first to know about any serious problems – not the last.

Chapter Eight

OLD PATTERNS DIE

ASSERTIVENESS

Assertiveness is about being able to make conscious choices about what to do for your highest good – in any given moment. Most people are drifters: they sleepwalk through their day and allow life to choose for them. This is a great shame, because being able to make conscious choices gives you enormous power – the power to create and direct your life, rather than role play your way through it. When you first start making conscious choices, you realize that there are only so many hours in a day, and that if you are to spend your day doing exactly what makes your heart sing, you must be selective. When you give yourself permission to do this, you are entering into a journey of self-discovery. You get to know yourself very quickly when you become conscious of the choices you make. The process of selecting this, over that, is empowering when you do it with awareness.

Another thing about assertiveness is that you can't do it part-time. To live assertively means you are making conscious choices across the board. This is a common blind spot for many women who believe, mistakenly, that if they are being assertive on one level, they must be being assertive on all of them – this doesn't hold. If, for example, you are honouring your choices at work, but crumble when it comes to relationships, then you are not living assertively. Assertiveness isn't about becoming overly defensive or aggressive either: if you are using force as a measure, it shows that you are struggling. And if you are struggling, then assertiveness has eluded you.

Assertiveness is not so much about *what* you do: it is about *how* you do it. Assertive high-flyers – those who have fine-tuned their assertiveness skills over time – have learnt to soften and bend because to them, the end, and the means, are the same. Out of this, they develop a loving contract with themselves. The choices that they make always reflect the tugging of their own heartstrings. They act, not out of selfishness, but out of a desire to live and let live. Anything less and you remain a drifter passively hitching a back seat ride, and letting life just happen to you.

Living assertively also includes taking care of your own personal safety. Unless you accept sole responsibility for your safety, you will never know what it feels like to be the one deciding where you are going, and how you will get there. Only by being the driver, and not the driven, can you find your power. Relying on the men close by to protect you is a sure way to lose your power – fathers, husbands, and brothers are often called on to rescue or champion a female's cause. If you can dare to take your personal safety into your own hands, you might be surprised at how much safer you feel. You might even decide that you don't need anyone else to watch your back – you are more than capable of doing it yourself. If you can fly in the face of the mainstream, and step out on your own, the courage you need to do it will find you.

Assertiveness is not about going to extremes, or about trying to control the world through aggression, or force. Assertiveness is about the law of appropriateness, and your ability to honour good judgement calls, most of the time. Once you have developed the wisdom to be firm when it is warranted, and gracious when it is deserved, it is incredible how little you need to do to get the result you want.

Assertiveness only works from the inside out. You can't become assertive by doing a weekend workshop in it, or by parroting what you have learnt from someone else. Of course, you have to start somewhere, and reading a book on it is a good place to begin. But at some point, you have to make what you have learnt your own. This means letting go of what others are telling you, putting the book down, and finding out the truth of it all for yourself. Once you do, the real work can start, and you will be on your way to understanding that true assertiveness is attained over time, through your own inner practice. It comes from the centre of you – your core – which always knows what course of action to take. It grows out of the softness within, and when you are eventually able to assert yourself on every level, you will know it. It won't feel like anything else you have ever done because, for the first time, *you* will be setting the pace. *You* will be the hub around which the wheel of life revolves.

My first job as a bouncer involved me practising some crowd control in one of Soho's busiest clubs. I stood in one place the entire night telling people where to go. I didn't need reminding how important it is to control the flow, and direction, of huge numbers of people in a large club. If an enormous volume of people gets out of control, there's very little you can do to alter its course. I didn't take my eye off the ball once. Every time someone was somewhere they weren't supposed to be, I'd ask them clearly, and politely, to move. I'd often pepper my exchanges with humour, which would put people at their ease. And using assertive body language made all the difference: I'd stand square and tall, but hold my arms open in a non-confrontational manner. People responded to this positively – they'd even herd themselves like sheep into a pen. When closing time came, the assistant manager of the club bounded up to me. "You've made quite an impact, Charly. We rarely have so few problems with crowd control. I love the way you operate: firm but fair, firm but fair. You are working tomorrow night, I hope?"

POUND FOR POUND

Don't defend by punching or kicking as it is unlikely that you will win this way. Pound for pound, you will probably not be able to punch as hard as a man. Even if you could, your attacker's arms are longer – he will reach you first. You are much better off saying goodbye to the pound for pound method of defence. It is, after all, only one way to defend out of so many. And look at what you are left with when you do: everything else.

It took me years as a martial artist to resist the temptation of using the pound for pound method of defence. For a long time, I thought I could win against anyone. Given the least opportunity, I would tit for tat my way out of any scrap. I would get hit and would hit back, and so it went with me charging at walls until one day, I realized that I didn't actually need to mirror what an opponent was doing: I could set my own rules.

While sparring at my next kick-boxing session, I put this to the test. My partner moved in quickly to strike to my head, but rather than play by the rules and defend with either a kick or a punch above the waist, I chose to break the pattern. A split second before his punch connected, I moved just an inch to the

side and turned to get behind him. I dropped down onto the back of his knee
with my full weight, and down he went, still swinging.

My partner was not a happy man after that. He later declared that I had, in fact,
lost our bout of sparring because I had broken the rules. I replied that in the real
world, there are no rules. Sometimes in order to survive, you have to go beyond
rules. The problem with the pound for pound method of defence is that it locks
you more deeply into them.

*It could be tedious on the doors on a quiet night: lots of standing around
and precious little to do. Sometimes my colleagues and I would rough-
house with each other to make the time go faster. One particular night, I
punched a colleague of mine on the arm – just as a joke. He was a big
Polish champion wrestler who had little idea of his own strength. He just
responded with the same – as a joke. The next move was interesting: as a
joke, we both threw a punch at the same time. His landed first, and it hurt.
I grew tired of these antics, which I usually lost. The next time we
scrapped, he threw another punch. This time, I dodged it. I shimmied to
the side as he moved forward, and pinched him in the ribs. He stayed away
from me after that.*

LINEAR THINKING

The assumption that only men can think in a straight line, and that women can
only mentally process intuitively, is a lie. Women have more nerve fibres in the
part of the brain that connects both hemispheres, which is why they are not only
able to use intuition and lateral thinking, but linear thinking also – should they
need to. It is a great advantage to be able to go at situations from almost any
angle. When it comes to staying safe, though, thinking only in the linear is
dangerous. The best defence against an attacker might not be to punch and kick
your way out of trouble, (the tit for tat strategy of defence is linear, like playing
tennis). The best you could do might be to think outside the box, and squirt
some Johnson's Baby Powder up your attacker's nose. Another option still,
might be to not retaliate at all, (there are times when your immediate
environment can help you out).

While linear thinking has its moments, it is important not to identify with it so
much that it keeps you stuck in a single groove. Life is an ever changing array
of different grooves, so to keep up, your think tank has got to be versatile and

flexible. Apart from anything, going at almost every problem in a straight line just isn't practical: acting like a ball bearing rolling down a single track keeps you blinkered and vulnerable. Most of all, it hinders communication – a bull charging at a matador is looking ahead, not to the sides. When people charge at trouble, a sideways push of information is usually not a consideration – as I was to find out one night.

A frantic message came over our radios shortly after we'd opened up one night. An incident was about to flare up between a couple on the dance floor: there might be carnage, and urgent backup was needed. Quick as a flash, five of my colleagues from outside jumped, sprung, leaped, and bounded into action. The heat was on, adrenalin levels were up, and without any clear idea of where they were going, or what they'd do when they got there, they flew through the inner doors and scattered to the four winds inside.

Twenty minutes later, a very irate head doorman walked out from inside. I overheard him speaking to his team over the radio. "The fight has dispersed on its own. No problem. I repeat, no problem on the dance floor. Everyone resume your positions. Oh, and – er, lads, next time a fight is about to kick off, can you please let us know where it is?"

DOING THE UNEXPECTED

To not do the expected is to connect profoundly with the power of the feminine. Feminine energy is like the wind. It blows this way and that, and can change direction at the drop of a hat. When you open to this power, you are free to flow in whatever way suits you best, in any given moment. Feminine power smashes through pattern: that is the reason why when it strikes, it seems to come out of nowhere. People rely on pattern; they like to know how things will begin, and how they will end. Without pattern, they have no guarantee; no control.

Not giving people what they are expecting means they can't read you. Become like the wind – it is its own master.

A street thug is an opportunist and has little time to set up an attack. If his target is a woman, he is banking on her reacting in the following way: she won't make fixed eye contact, she will probably be passive, and she will almost certainly be hesitant. Instead of letting an attacker surprise you, why not surprise him? Face him square on, make unswerving eye contact, and stand bold and sure to your boots. Doing this brings much more power into the mix than you might suspect: your attacker is expecting this reaction from a man, not a woman.

Not doing what you are supposed to will present an attacker with a contradiction. This will not only slow him down, it might also persuade him to reconsider: if you are defiant enough not to respond in the way that you should, what else are you capable of?

I fast developed a reputation as a maverick while on the doors. No one could ever be sure how I'd react to anything. I could be calm and cool-headed one minute, then hurling some angry lout out through the doors the next. You could say I was either respected or vilified by my colleagues: an unpredictable woman at best, and a breaker of sacred gender law at worst. A lot of male feathers got ruffled when I was around. There was a pay-off, though, for not doing what my fellow bouncers expected. I got to be authentic, moment to moment, and there is power in that.

A man once walked in through the doors, took one look at me, and said, "Ooh! A female bouncer! Ooh! Being frisked by a woman—lovely—corr—some of that!"

I courteously waved the man over. With tongue hanging out and pelvis forward, he shuffled over for what he thought would be a bit of touchy feely. His dream of being searched by a female bouncer had at last come true. As he stood panting like a bloodhound, with arms up and legs apart, I gently frisked him everywhere – a little too well. The man dropped to his knees clutching his groin. He was putty in my hands after that.

SLOWING DOWN TO SPEED UP

If you are attacked, resist the temptation of responding with a frantic and undirected defence. Instead, slow down your mind and body. When the time is right, you will reply with appropriate action. A well considered, and measured defence, will serve you more effectively, and faster, than a hasty one.

Don't assume the worst if you are ever in serious danger. Bear in mind that if an attacker intends to rape you, you usually have more time to work out a defence than you imagine. It is physically impossible, for example, for a man to rape you if his zip is still done up. In order to unzip himself, he must release one hand he is holding you with, to do it. There is often a window of opportunity here to defend and get away. In most rape attacks, there is usually at least one opportunity to defend yourself, but you will only see this opening if you stay calm enough. If you can just keep your terror under control and watch things as they unfold, step by step, your chances of survival are so much greater. And this way, when you do eventually defend, it will count. Timing is everything: if you strike too early, you might not live to regret it.

The inexperienced rush into danger: all they need to justify their haste is a target. Those who have learnt from experience pull back for a moment to assess what they can't see, as well as what they can. I applied this truth one night when I was running the doors at a large nightclub in central London. The head doorman had asked me to take over from him for the night – he had a mission of mercy to deal with in another part of town. I stepped up to the challenge like a trooper, and leapt at the chance of running the doors my way. With no real system in place for keeping the peace, it was always panic stations when he was around. His bouncers were more like loose bits of shrapnel all firing off in different directions, rather than a tight, organized team. They'd all flounder in a puddle of confusion, and end up creating far more problems than they ever solved. It wasn't difficult to see why: they hardly ever spoke to each other over their radios. The only time they did, was just after trouble had erupted. It never occurred to them that regularly checking in with each other might prevent violence from starting. Yes. It was time to have a go at doing things my way. One night was all I needed to whip the talented, but aimless team into shape. I had no doubt in my mind that in that time, I could bring order to chaos. I also had faith that my shot at leadership would greatly increase my colleagues' chances of staying in one piece.
I tackled the job with military precision by making sure that every bouncer knew what his job was, and where he was supposed to be stationed. I

opened the lines of communication – knowledge is always power when it comes to safety. I also made a new ground rule: no one was to single-handedly jump in to sort out trouble – my colleagues had so often done this with disastrous consequences. And last, but not least, I made it clear that not one bouncer was to move unless I gave the go-ahead, and was satisfied that adequate backup was in place.

A few hours into the shift, I had them operating as a single unit. They'd grown into such a slick team of operators that when trouble first hit, every one of them held back. They waited just long enough for me to tell them where, when, and whom, and only then did they spring into action. The upshot was that while my colleagues were a fraction slower to deal with any trouble, they were always faster to sort it out.

I was known on the doors as a "master searcher". Managers of some of the clubs I worked at would often place me just inside the front door early on in the evening, to search people as they entered – drugs, alcohol, and weapons were not permitted in these places. I was valuable as I managed to stop more non-permitted items coming in through the front door than most of my colleagues. We were all briefed on how best to do the job: no familiarities, no polite conversation – just frisk and move on to the next.

I had my own ideas. My strategy involved going directly against what I'd been told to do. I'd take my time, and I'd greet and chat to the people I was searching – I wouldn't be rushed. Searching this way had its upside: I made many of the clubbers I was frisking feel so relaxed, that they'd often trip themselves up by letting slip information that they later regretted – bottles, knives, and weed wouldn't be hard to find. I'd also make a point of listening to each clubber as I searched them: paying close attention to someone's voice is often a reliable way of judging sobriety.

Doing the opposite of what I'd been told to do, however, didn't go down well with everyone. One night, the manager of the venue I happened to be working at dragged me into his office and laid into me for not searching faster than I was.

"Charly!" he roared, "I've told you before to f—g 'urry up with the searchin'! We've gotta get people in faster. You're slowin' us down!"

"Actually," I answered, "I think I'm speeding you up. Have you any idea what's in a handshake?"

The manager despised anyone cleverer than him, but he despised a lack of professionalism even more.

"Get out of 'ere!" he growled. "And f—g do your job!"

I never heard a peep out of him after that. From that night on, he let me do things my way – reluctantly.

THE ELEMENT OF SURPRISE

Having the element of surprise in your arsenal of safety tools is a huge advantage. It is one of those things that everyone knows about, but few ever take seriously. The fact is, using any element of surprise can be the difference between life and death. You come out of a supermarket and an attacker pounces as you are putting all your shopping into the boot of your car. You grab the frozen leg of lamb from your shopping bag, and whack him in the face with it. You follow up with a lightning fast uppercut to his chin with a tin of pork luncheon meat. You then finish him off with a sharp jab to his gonads with a courgette. Your attacker is now in a quandary, because you have robbed him of three things: initiative, rhythm, and control.

One of the best ways to see the element of surprise in action, is in supermarkets. Watch what happens when you take all your groceries to the till, and tell the person totting them all up that you don't want a receipt. They will nod and hear your request, but as they hand you your change, they will give you a receipt anyway. When you hand it back saying that you did ask them not to give it to you in the first place, they will glare at you as if you have just attacked them with a machete. You have interrupted their flow and rhythm, and they freeze, just for a moment.

When you throw the element of surprise into situations, you create a momentary glitch. There is protection to be had in a momentary glitch.

When young men insisted on wearing their jeans hanging below their buttocks, I'd always be tempted to call their bluff. One night, a group of homies walked in and after being searched, they all stood vacantly around in the reception area, waiting for their pre-booked tickets. I was of a mind to reinforce the club's dress code using humour, rather than the heavy-duty approach I'd been instructed to use. I crept up behind the tallest youngster, who was leaning against the ticket desk showing himself in all

his glory, and yanked his trousers right down to his ankles. A whole lobby of clubbers, staff, and bouncers witnessed the spectacle: stick thin legs poking out from beneath the longest and baggiest boxer shorts you can imagine – it was a picture.

The horrified youngster dropped like a plumb weight to gather his trousers, as well as his pride. "What did you do that for?" he shrieked.

"Well," I replied, "your trousers were so low down, that I assumed you wanted them off."

There is a point to all this: the boy was a well known troublemaker, and was allowed in on the understanding that he behave – even so much as a stare in the wrong direction and he'd be out. Pulling his trousers down had been a surprise of the worst kind for him, but it did serve a purpose: the young lad behaved impeccably the entire night. Every time he saw me coming, he clutched his trouser belt and delivered a nervous cackle. I suppose not having his slender legs exposed was more important than causing trouble.

The greatest martial arts teacher I ever had was a powerful, hard as nails bloke who trained men to go out and fight in Afghanistan. In order to earn my diploma as a teacher of personal protection, I had to have a one-on-one session with him in a squash court: he'd play the part of some thug in one of the clubs I was working in, and I'd have to throw him out through the squash court door. He'd attack, and I'd defend – that was the plan.

At first, things seemed to be chugging along well enough. I'd remembered most of what he'd taught me and was more than able to hold my own each time he attacked. Near the end of the session, however, the atmosphere became tense when my coach suddenly morphed into all the violent louts that I'd ever encountered over my years on the doors. No more mister nice guy: it was either do, or get hurt. As fast as a flick of a switch, my mood changed. Realizing that this was no longer a learning curve, I quietened down, stood stock-still, and waited nervously in the middle of the room for my teacher's next move. With the speed of a tornado, and with more aggression than I was prepared for, he lunged at me from behind and grabbed me in a bear hug. Using a technique he'd taught me, I just managed to swivel round so that I was behind him. Using one hand, I got hold of his shorts at the front and twisted them into a knot, putting

*pressure on his groin, and with my other arm secured a tight headlock –
and kept it on. It was time to shove him out through the door. I pushed, I
strained, I tore every muscle to get him to inch towards the door, but the
man was immovable; he just wouldn't shift and for the first time, I
panicked. I was only too aware that getting my diploma depended on me
hauling my coach out through the squash court door. I just couldn't
entertain the possibility of failing to get it – I'd trained so hard. I'd
endured years of battered limbs, and purple bruises the size of dinner
plates. No. I wasn't going to let all this slip through my fingers. I'd pull
one out of the bag, somehow.*

*What happened next shook me: I found myself in a place of absolutely no
doubt. It's the kind of feeling you get when every part of you just knows
something beyond thinking or hesitation. It's the kind of feeling that gives
you the audacity to do something completely left-field. In a state of altered
consciousness, I squeezed my coach's shorts at the front even tighter,
released the headlock, and with my free hand reached down at the back
and rammed my fingers into his buttocks. As if he'd been stung on the
bottom by a bee, my coach howled, arched backwards, and, with arms
flying, shuffled onto the tips of his toes. Out through the door he went, all
fourteen stone of him – hips first.*

*Days later, I got my diploma. My coach shared a few discreet words as he
handed it to me. "Charly, you've earned your stripes. By the way," he
continued, clearing his throat, "that was a neat move you made near the
end of the session. Yeah. Never saw that one coming."*

Chapter Nine

POWER TO THE WOMEN

FEMININE POWER

When water destroys, it does so without warning. A tsunami strikes with an immediacy that is hard to comprehend: a wall of water rises out of the ocean and, with the speed of a jet plane, silently moves towards land. It is merciless and ferocious; it is unstoppable. Feminine power can be like this. If you feel your safety might be compromised in any way, defend without warning. It will seem to your attacker that your defence came out of nowhere, like a tsunami.

Feminine power is always being underestimated. Whether you find yourself in a battle of words or fists, your ability to protect yourself will always be questionable, to a male attacker. Don't feel bad about being taken for granted, but instead applaud it as you can use this to your advantage. Your attacker will almost certainly not be using as much force to overpower you as he would a man. He will be taking it as an article of faith that you are much weaker than he is. Because of this, he will be so puffed up with complacency that he will become overconfident about the outcome – as far as he is concerned, there is no way that you can win. Have you ever noticed that the more air you blow into a balloon, the easier it is to make it go pop?

Shortly before closing time one night, a stocky Polish bouncer I'd been working with decided to have a bit of fun – at my expense. It had been a quiet night, and my excitable colleague still had a lot of energy to burn. He ducked down low, stamped his foot like a bull about to charge, and launched himself towards me. Not thinking for a moment that he was serious, I just stood there like a rabbit caught in headlights and watched him close in. Before I knew where I was, he'd got me in a fireman's lift

and was bouncing me up and down in the air like a performing chimp.
"Put me down!" I shouted.
"What can you do?" he answered. "Nothing! You are only a woman!"
My Polish colleague ignored my demand, pinned me securely against his
shoulder, and spun around like a whirling dervish.
I went with the flow and played along for a bit, but a few spins into the
scrap and I'd had enough. My Polish colleague was now holding me
firmly with both arms, and had no intention of putting me down. To my
way of thinking, that gave me the right to do whatever it took to get him to
put me down. Without a second thought, I cupped both hands and smacked
them quickly, but lightly, over his ears. Disorientated and giddy, the burly
Pole staggered to the four cardinal directions, covered his ears with his
palms, and swore at me for hurting his eardrums. Down I went like a ton
of bricks – a somewhat bumpy victory, but a victory nonetheless.

INGENUITY OVER BRAWN

Most women assume that if they are attacked by a man, the man will win.
Actually, that is a complete fallacy. If a small man can defeat a much bigger
one, then so can you. It is all about using ingenuity. As a woman, you have bags
of that, but only once you pull away from trying to solve things with muscle.
Most attackers rely solely on their physical strength to overpower you. You
can't win against a predator who is brawn led – he has much more of it than
you do. But ingenuity is something that you have much more of than he does.
You just need to concentrate on being creative, rather than reactive.

I was in a dojo once practising some ju-jitsu grappling drills with a man who
was enormously strong. The sensei, in his wisdom, had paired us up. As I stood
on the mat waiting for the signal to start, I gawped at my partner's considerable
bulk and felt an immediate terror-induced rush of adrenalin. A vision of me
ending up underneath, what looked like, over fifteen stone of prize beef, almost
had me conceding defeat before the tussle had even begun. That day,
determination was stronger than fear. I steadied my nerves, and waited. Without
warning, my muscle-bound partner suddenly ducked down and lunged. Before
he was able to get me in a front bear hug, I crouched down even lower, lunged
towards him, and landed in a bellyflop, with my arms tightly locked around his
ankle. With my entire body weight, I pushed forward into his lower leg, and
down he went with a smack. To make sure he stayed down, I sprawled all over
him, twisted his wrist into a tight lock, and pressed my elbow against his ear.
The over fifteen-stoner wriggled and fought to break free like a fish caught in a

net. That was my first experience of defending creatively, rather than reactively. I haven't sweated the big stuff since.

There is no need to get into victim mode if you are having a difficult time getting rid of unwanted male attention – there is plenty you can do. If a man is really becoming a nuisance, you can very gently step on his foot with your stiletto – that will make him take a few steps back. You then apologize profusely, and he will understand as you did it quite by accident. If that doesn't work, try this: politely explain that you are feeling violently sick. If your pursuer is still not taking the hint, put your hand over your mouth as if you are about to vomit, then rush to the ladies' powder room. Trust me, when you come out, he won't be waiting.

A steady stream of excitable clubbers all out to have a blast piled in through the doors of one of north London's busiest nightclubs. It was peak time on a Saturday night, and I'd been told to stand downstairs by the biggest dance floor to keep all walkways clear for clubbers to circulate through. Good traffic control inside a hectic nightclub is a serious security issue: if enough people squeeze into a tiny area, at best, tempers will rise and at worst, you have a riot on your hands. I did manage to keep all of the main arteries clear for some while – that was until two stocky men with beer glasses plonked themselves close to the dance floor, right in the middle of a major route. Clubbers were now having trouble getting from one side of the club to the other, and a bottleneck was in the making. "Charly, people can't move down there," said the head doorman, watching goings-on downstairs on a camera by the front door. "Clear the place will you, before it becomes a safety hazard."

The two beer-swillers would have to go. As I walked towards them, I could see that getting them to move might present a challenge: two alpha males eyeing up a couple of pretty young things – a juggernaut wouldn't have shifted them. Knowing that the head doorman upstairs was watching my every move, I did things by the book and politely asked the two beer-swillers to move elsewhere. They didn't speak, but just looked at me. It was a look I'd seen once too often from men who considered themselves far too important to take any notice of a female bouncer. They waved me away like a couple of courtiers dismissing a serving wench, and told me to go and make life miserable for someone else.

The next thing I did was a first: instead of calling for backup, I hesitated. While I knew that the head doorman upstairs was relying on me to sort the area, and would be down in a heartbeat if needed, I also knew that I could get the two beer-swillers to move on my own. While I was deciding on the best way to do it, I happened to notice a man taking a great deal of interest in the two of them from the other side of the dance floor. He was clearly ogling them both, and made no secret of the fact. I wandered over to the man to find out more.

"Ooh! I fancy the pants off of one of them," he sighed, tightly pursing his lips together. "That one on the left with the cheeky smile," he continued, pointing him out with a well groomed pinky.

"The one with the cheeky smile has been trying to get your attention for a while now," I said, injecting as much enthusiasm as I could to feed the gay man's already all-consuming lust. "I think he's really ke—"

Before I'd even finished talking, the gay man was off. With a high fashion strut and a Polo Mint pout, he cleared the dance floor faster than anyone had any right to, and began the chase. Just as he was about to address the object of his desire, the two beer-swillers took one look at him, dropped their beers, and ran for the exit.

FEMININE GIFTS

It is hard for many women to push past the assumption that only men can keep them safe. Actually, you can take care of your own personal safety much more effectively by using the feminine gifts that you have in abundance – even when things get physical. The belief that muscle power alone is the answer to physical attack is to sell yourself short: you have more resources to rely on than you imagine. The feminine gift of intuition, for example, is one of your most powerful allies. Intuition is higher intelligence, and when you use it, you are tapping into a vast, invisible reservoir of information that most people don't know exists. When the world around you tells you to do this, you do that, because you have intuition on your side; you have higher knowledge guiding you.

A sophisticated grasp of timing is another feminine gift you can rely on – timing is everything. When making a decision, how often have you allowed your inner clock to advise you? Try and remember how it felt to hear that almost imperceptible inner voice whisper that the time isn't right yet – maybe tomorrow, maybe in a year, but not now. When you allow your inner clock to set the pace, you are claiming full responsibility for your own life – personal safety included.

The feminine ability to see relationships in all things can, at the highest level, take you to the divine. Women are hardwired for recognizing and making connections and, as mentioned earlier, have a far more integrated cerebral make-up. Their capacity for both intuition and logic is the reason why they see whole pictures, rather than just parts of them. Seeing things whole gives you two things: it gives you more information to play with, and it enables you to see the origin of pathological behaviour – the shadow is invisible to most.

Another gift of femininity is the ability to experience life across, rather than as hierarchical. Dealing with danger when you aren't looking up or down becomes a much more practical affair: if danger strikes, allies are never too far out of reach because they are on the same level.

To be feminine *is* to be gifted, for femininity holds such riches. Find these riches, dig them up, and see what they can do for you. I did, and I was always two steps ahead of any danger. If trouble did ever strike, it always arrived late – for me.

The Void, or the great mystery, is also a gift of femininity. The Void is a gift because she is there. She is an inner, timeless place that women are aware of, consciously or not. The Void is often referred to as the Great Nothing, but I prefer to call her the Great Everything, for she is the hidden cave of infinite possibility; she is the invisible womb and generator of all potential.

The Great Everything is feminine in nature because she is the hidden counterpart to the masculine world of form. We can only know ourselves at root by going through her first. You won't be able to go the distance, though, if you are carrying excess baggage – you need every bit of energy to withstand the unknown. Travelling into the Void is the same as travelling to the centre of you. If you are to get there, you must ditch all the beliefs that have come to you from the outside. You will have to bag all the labels that the world has slapped on you from birth – within, as well as without.

If you can hack it, there is everything to be gained because no longer having any secrets frees up enormous energy. In the film, *The Matrix*, Neo can only touch his power once he knows who he truly is. When he goes to see the Oracle, she explains that unless he can clearly see every aspect of himself, he cannot become whole; he cannot become the "One". She points to a sign on the wall above the doorway: "Know thyself".

Long ago, you slammed room doors shut and threw away the key. The Void can help you find those rooms again. She can help you reopen them, and pull off the dust sheets of buried potential. All those experiences that you pushed into obscurity hold so much latent energy. Journeying to the Void will feel like travelling blind; it will feel as if you have lost all points of reference. But that is the point: you can only find new points of reference once you have dropped the old ones.

Looking your true self in the eye not only unlocks vast reserves of energy and power, it also keeps you safe. Extra power brings with it a much more integrated relationship with the world: if danger should ever tap you on the shoulder, chances are you will be ready.

Early on as a martial artist, I always kept an open mind as to what my abilities in the physical department were. More often than not, martial arts teachers would make assumptions about my strength in order to undermine my physical power. The physical standard of "inequality" between the sexes had to be maintained – it was simpler that way. Not making the same assumptions about my physical potential was a smart thing to do because I got to find out, first-hand, what I was capable of. In no time, I had graduated from lifting someone two stone heavier than me, to taking over twenty stone on my back.

When you make assumptions about your physical strength you give away your power. Never collude with someone else's expectations. Women, after all, have been known to lift cars single-handedly when trying to save a child trapped underneath. How were they able to do this? In a moment of great need, they connected to a power that comes from an invisible place. They opened to a force that is both within, and without. In this way, they defied all worldly expectations and made the impossible, possible.

Practical jokes are all very well but when you are the joke, things suddenly don't seem quite so amusing. One night, a colleague I was working with called me to an exit at the back of the club. A drunken man had collapsed at the top of the staircase and needed to be ejected immediately. When I got to the exit, three colleagues were standing over one of the most enormous men I'd ever seen. The oversized clubber cast quite a shadow as

he lay on his back, purring like a big cat.

"Okay, lads," I said, clicking my fingers, "this should be easy work between the four of us." I knelt down, grabbed a chubby arm, and got stuck in. I loved teamwork. You can achieve anything when everyone pitches in – you can move a mountain.

With gusto, I plunged in and lost myself to the moment so entirely, that I failed to notice that I was the only one doing anything. It was only when I looked up to offer a sensible strategy for moving the heavyweight, that I saw my colleagues all huddled together in a corner, basking in a private bit of tittering.

"Er – we're off, Charly," said one of them, straining so hard to stifle his giggles that he pretended he was crying. "Some bloke at the bar is spark out. You won't have any problem getting snoozy here outside. You're tough!" With that, they roared with uncontrollable laughter, and left.

There I was, alone and lumbered with the task of having to move almost thirty stone of dead weight to the back door, which was roughly ten yards away. I leant back against the wall and quietly sighed. I hated being set up, and it was plain to see that the last laugh would be on me – or would it?

Twenty minutes later, my colleagues were burning with curiosity about developments at the back exit. "Charly! You still trying to move that huge lump of a guy at the back door?"

I paused before stealing their thunder. "He's out. I've been back at the front door now for the last ten minutes. You got any more heavyweights to eject?"

They ran, they raced, they shot through the dance floor and were with me before I could say three blind mice. "Did you really get that geezer out?" they all asked at once.

"Go and see for yourself," I said, coolly. "He's lying on the pavement next to the Tesco trolley bank, whistling in his sleep."

My colleagues fell into a tight scrum and hatched a plot. One of them shot off towards the back exit to check out my story, and in a trice was back looking ashen. "Stone me! How'd you do it?" he asked, looking me up and down to make quite sure I was made of flesh and bone. "Us lot would've had trouble between the three of us!"

All three stared at the floor to mask the humiliation of having been outsmarted. How I'd got the better of them would, and shall, remain a secret. They didn't need to know what had really happened: that I'd spotted a very slippery, long plastic mat next to the unconscious heavyweight on the floor. And that I managed to roll him onto it and drag him, in less than ten minutes, all the way to the back door before putting him out to pasture. No. They really didn't need to know that.

PUTTING OUT SMALL FIRES

The female warrior focusses on little things because she knows that they can lead to big things. Putting out a small fire, for example, will prevent a large one from starting. It occurs to me that all the little things are not so little, and that dealing with all small fires keeps you safe. When you stamp out the faintest flicker of danger, nothing ever gets too big to handle.

Many of the bouncers I worked with didn't see it as their job to take responsibility for nipping trouble in the bud. They were there to sort out violence after the fact. I, on the other hand, considered it essential to put a stop to the earliest signs of trouble – that was my speciality. I'd keep things tidy by putting out as many small fires as I could. A small fire could be anything from disgruntled drinkers arguing with bar staff over money, to women being chased up and down the dance floor by men only too eager to undo their zips. In my view, if enough of us on the doors concentrated on putting out any small fires, we'd have very few big ones to contend with – if any.

While patrolling a crowded dance floor one night, the hairs on the back of my neck stood up – I knew a fight was brewing. I became very present, and watched. Sure enough, two well oiled lads parked near the centre of the dance floor started sizing each other up. Just as they were about to close in for a punch-up, I radioed my colleague over on the other side of the floor. "Darren, something's about to flare up on the dance floor to your right. Meet me there." I followed the shouting to the middle of the dance floor and waited, but my colleague never showed. I radioed him again – no response. Alone, and eager to stop a fight before it had even begun, I took a risk and single-handedly jumped in to stop the two young hotheads from pulverizing each other. Luckily for me, the two lads were more talk than action, and after gentle persuasion, agreed to shake hands and go their separate ways.

Relieved that I'd stopped a small fire from becoming a much bigger one, I turned my attention to finding out why my colleague hadn't answered his radio and joined me on the dance floor. When I caught up with him, he was propped up against a door frame sleeping like a baby – the man was as much good as a toy Action Man.

At the end of the night, I confronted my dopey colleague and had it out with him. I put it to him that although the two lads I'd pulled apart hadn't quite gone the distance and exchanged blows, it was still reason enough to be on the alert. My lackadaisical colleague thought the whole incident was a storm in a teacup. "Charly, nothin' 'appened," he said defensively, yawning so hard that I could've fitted my head in his mouth with room to spare. "I'm 'ere to deal with a fight that's already started. I'm not gonna move 'cause people are bad-mouthin' each other," he continued, rubbing his eyes. "That's not what I call trouble!"

With that, he stared in my direction as if in a dream, and slowly ambled back to his station by the door. I suppose the only thing that would've kept the man awake while on the job was a big fire. I hope he managed to find one. I didn't stay around long enough to find out. I found another club to work at where they preferred small fires, to big ones.

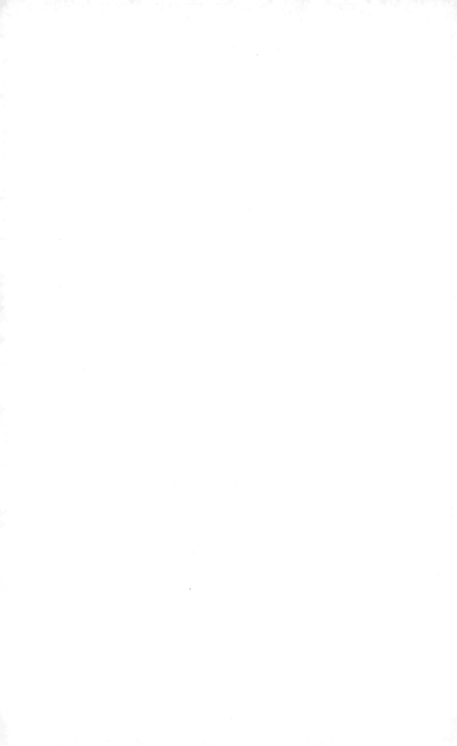

Chapter Ten

I CAN SEE EVERYTHING FROM IN HERE!

ENERGY

Everything boils down to energy. There are really only two kinds of it: visible and invisible. Visible energy is physical: how hard must you twist the lid of a jar to open it? How much effort must you apply when pushing your broken-down car to the nearest garage? Invisible energy, by contrast, is subtle. You can't see it, but it is there all the same – it lies at the heart of everything. Without invisible energy, there is no physical energy – the visible is born of the invisible. A punch, therefore, has no way of knowing where, how fast, or how hard, without the command from the invisible place.

Thoughts and feelings come from the invisible place – the subtle – and your outer world is constantly being shaped by them. Do your own research and watch how the world around you responds to each feeling and thought that you have. Notice how the outside world begins to mirror your internal landscape. Once you awaken to the realization that your inner space influences your outer space, you can create whatever circumstance you desire. If it is safety you crave, it is safety you can have – from the inside out.

When we express energy through *doing,* and we interpret success, on every level, as the sum total of our actions, then we are applying the masculine principle. The masculine principle is defined by what it has, and what it does. It manifests through external force. When defending against an attack, you have the choice to either block, or strike, or run.

If, by contrast, you are living a life that is directed from within, then you are energetically aligned to the way of the feminine. The feminine principle is expressed through *being.* It is an inner state that finds meaning through non-action. The feminine principle has no overt measure for success, because *being,* and *experiencing,* are their own reward. Feminine energy is the reason and intent behind all external action. Aligning to it makes it possible to pre-empt any potential danger coming at us from the world of form. If we open to feminine energy, we never need block, or strike, or run.

It was my first night at a new club, and the head doorman decided to put me just inside the front door for the night, to see how I got on. The club was full to bursting and he was nervous about putting a woman on normal dance floor duty – the last thing he wanted was a female bouncer getting hurt. If I'd been a man, this consideration wouldn't have been offered, but the men I was working with that night were "iron-pumpers" of the chunkiest kind – with egos to match. In their world, boys were boys and girls had to be, well, dependent. While I'd always forced myself to bite the bullet where chauvinism was concerned, that night the head doorman's obvious lack of trust in my abilities as a female bouncer was making me fume – and it showed. This particular head doorman, however, was wise enough to know that a happy team was a more efficient team: he was quick to notice my frustration, and allowed me to walk around inside later on.

The head doorman's decision to move me from the front door to the interior was auspicious because it enabled me to experience something I'd only ever felt once before: fearlessness. As I patrolled inside, I took in all the new sounds, smells, and sights of the place, and I marvelled at my lack of any first night nerves, or concern for what ifs. An invisible siphon had sucked every last vestige of self-doubt out of me, and left an unshakable belief in my ability to handle anything – no matter how dangerous. I basked in that feeling and settled into an easy, comfortable stride as I watched over the crowd.

It's a wonderful thing to be without fear when you're surrounded with danger. Only when you're fearless can you properly witness the effect you are having on the external world. That night, I had a first glimpse of how responsive the outer world can be to an inner state. As people approached, I noticed that they were responding in a way they never had before: they'd size me up before coming anywhere near, and would hesitate before asking me something. They'd also keep moving out of my way in an effort to give me more room to pass.

After a whole evening of this, I realized that not holding fear was making people tense. I mulled it all over right up until closing time. As the head doorman and I stood holding open the front doors for any last stragglers, a slightly merry young man wandered up to my colleague, slapped him on the shoulder, and said, "Blimey, mate, she's scarier than you are!"

Nature abhors a vacuum. If fear has moved out, its opposite takes up residence – love. Love is an energy that connects you to real power. Once you've traded in fear for love, you project a completely different kind of energy. People will pick up on that energy, subliminally, but because most are fear-based, it will make them nervous. Love is an awesome force – far too immense for most to either recognize, or hold.

THE VOID

We can't see the Void, but we can, on occasion, feel her presence – if we are lucky. Respecting the Void is to be comfortable with not having to have an answer. This is a powerful tool for staying safe because when you are content with not having to know what an attacker will do, you have no more need to anticipate. This means you are far more likely to survive whatever attack comes at you. Not having to know *what isn't* happening, helps you survive *what is*.

Because the Void contains within her all potential, you have unlimited choice – at any given moment – of what to do for your highest good. The Void silently lies in wait, and if you have the courage to invite her in, she will guide you on every level. Your safety becomes a matter of trust: you make a choice, you act on it, and the Void takes care of the outcome.

I'd just opened the front doors one night, and was standing outside on the pavement waiting for my team to arrive: they were late, I was on my own, and I couldn't have been less worried. I was in a philosophical mood. I felt relaxed, and at ease. Just as I was enjoying a rare moment of stillness outside, the manager's pimply face popped out from behind the front door. "Charly, dark blue coat, middle-aged, nursing a pint at the bar: chuck him out. He's tight!" I walked inside and after a few words with the man, it was

obvious that he wasn't. I was reluctant to throw someone out for little reason, but for no reason at all... I decided to let it go.

A while later, the manager had another go at me and this time came outside to make his point. "Charly, what's the matter with you? Do your job and get that f—g idiot out! He's had enough!"

"No – he – hasn't!" I snapped. "Unless he's prancing around on the stage doing a pole dance in the buff, he stays put!"

The manager cursed under his breath and stormed back inside. At last, I was alone and left in peace to snatch a few more precious minutes of calm before the usual rush. With my back to the front door, I let my mind drift away from the stark world of club land. As the last of a recent downpour trickled down rooftops and pavement gutters, I meditated on the lamplight reflected in the grey, rain-filled cobblestones in the road. I gazed into moonlit puddles that danced and rippled in a gentle breeze. The beauty of it all, set against the ugliness of the world behind me, was almost too much to bear – a contrast that pinched at my soul like a spike. Sooner or later, I knew I'd have to choose between beauty and ugliness. The breeze outside was now picking up. Empty beer bottles blown from a nearby dumpster playfully rolled out of sight, tinkling like a wind chime as they faded – beauty was inescapable. I wondered if she was tenderly nudging me into seeing that I had already chosen her. It was true that once I'd always been only too eager to use violence – if the chance arose. Could I have crossed over from ugliness without even realizing it? The only thing I yearned for that night, in that place, was for beauty to take charge, and open the way to a higher power. Perhaps beauty had claimed me after all...

"Charly!" yelled the manager from inside the doorway. "If you don't sling that a—e out, I don't want you back!" Not even the badgering of a spotty, crimson-faced manager could galvanize me into action. Even the prospect of losing my job couldn't extinguish an overwhelming trust that things would just work out.

Half an hour later, though, I thought better of risking another bout of nagging from the manager. In order to keep the peace, as well as hold onto my job, I wandered inside to at least go through the motions of showing the man to the door – a token gesture to show willing. I tapped the man on the shoulder and very politely asked him to leave. He responded just as I thought he would: he wouldn't move unless "he decided to", and he'd take as long as he "bloody well wanted to". I asked the man a second time to make his way out, but he just sneered and carried on guzzling. Even at this point, getting physical didn't appeal. It was as if I was waiting for something.

The manager was now glowering at me from behind the bar. "Charly! Get the w—r out! Either he goes, or you do!"

I'd finally had enough. I'd waited long enough for some force from on high to help me out of all this – it was time to do some bouncing. I switched myself into action mode, went to grab the troublemaker, but just as I did, a colossal brute of a man sprung from a smoky corner of the dance floor, and lunged towards him. "You t—r! You're the bloke I've been looking for! I wanna word with you, mate – outside!"

The man I was about to throw out was lifted up by his lapels, thrown over the much bigger man's muscular shoulder like a two kilogramme dumb-bell, and carted out.

PERCEPTION

You can't protect yourself without developing perception. To perceive danger looming, you have to fine-tune your senses. This is not an easy thing to do as humans are trained, from birth, to be blinkered; they are domesticated into seeing with tunnel vision. As soon as people are born, primary indoctrination begins: parents regurgitate and force-feed a way of seeing that they were taught. As people grow up, the world around them takes over, and secondary indoctrination steps in. The education, fashion, health, and media industries all conspire to cement, and hypnotize, the collective gaze.

Accepting as an article of faith that an event you are witnessing is only part of a bigger one, is the first step to opening up your senses. It is a question of understanding that there are other things happening around that event that could be contributing to it – or even causing it. To begin to see with your senses you must agree to be different, and not swallow what the guiding forces in the world are trying so hard to make you believe: that what is unfolding in front of you is all there is.

Developing, and heightening perception, is a bit like having surround sound available to you. Some women and men of power have such sharp senses, that they have three hundred and sixty degree vision; they are walking lighthouse beacons that can home in on any potential danger way in the distance.

It is possible to fine-tune your senses to that degree, and use them to perceive the world as it is, rather than as it appears.

Great martial arts teachers have such acute senses that they can feel you approach from behind. They register a minute disturbance in the air around them, as your body moves through it. You too have the ability to do this: if you just remain still, really listen, and keep watching, you can learn to sense the earliest sign of danger from the subtle world. Practise putting your ear to the ground next time a storm is on the way. If you listen hard, you will be able to both hear, and feel, the faint roar of distant thunder in the earth well before you hear it in the sky.

Animals are masters at perceiving danger before it manifests. If the wind is blowing their way, they will smell you before they can see you. Watching animals can be a reliable way of knowing whether you are safe or not. Think of all the birds and fish that flee land and sea before a tsunami hits. If you are still around after they have left, it might be wise to leave the area – sharpish.

Have you ever wondered why magicians loathe showing tricks to children? Children are always looking where they shouldn't. Actually, they are always looking where they should because they focus on what isn't happening, as well as what is. A group of toddlers watches a magician hide a white rabbit, but little Tabatha is far more interested in checking out the underside of the magician's table. This is why she knows exactly what has happened to the white rabbit: her eyes have not only been looking at the white rabbit, but at everything else too.

Spend a day noticing everything that isn't happening, as well as everything that is. When someone speaks to you, don't focus only on them: take in their surroundings too. You know the man you are chatting to is with a friend: watch him as well – you can tell a great deal about someone by the company they keep. Notice the friend pouring something into a woman's drink at the bar: re-evaluate your situation and ask yourself if you really want to be there. As you shake a stranger's hand, be aware of where his other hand is: unconsciously, when people greet you with only one hand visible, they often have something to hide.

Look out at the world with a child's eyes. Become a walking sponge, and perceive the world in its entirety, like children do. Tabatha would tell you as much. That was, after all, the way she learnt to tell the difference between reality, and illusion.

It was near closing time at one of London's most popular watering holes and nerves were on edge. Irritable clubbers jostled for space as they waited to pick up their coats from the cloakroom before leaving. I was hovering nearby, gently trying to talk people into getting in line, when one of the cloakroom boys was attacked – right in front of me. A man who'd been drinking at the bar for most of the night swung for the fragile-looking member of staff. Before he had time to use his fist again, five bulked up doormen leaped out of the blackness and dragged him to the floor. Alcohol and drugs had made the man three times as strong, and three times as hard to restrain – getting him down was one thing, but keeping him down was quite another.

The violent clubber had a major grudge: when he'd gone to the cloakroom to get his coat, the cloakroom boy couldn't find it. After twenty minutes the coat still couldn't be found, and by this time the man's temper had reached boiling point. When he tried to get the cloakroom boy to admit that he'd lost it, the lad buckled, went to jelly, and tried to fob him off with vagueness and excuses. A powerful jab to the lad's jaw followed, which luckily only just connected.

The violent clubber was now gaining strength and was still intoxicated enough to comfortably take on five doormen. As he lashed out with fists, feet, and teeth, I saw something in my colleagues that I'd never seen before: doubt.

During all this, I did something that I'd trained myself to do in dangerous situations: I softened my gaze, allowed my eyes to wander away from all the drama at my feet, and tried to notice anything helpful from the unobvious further away. I suddenly found myself watching a man who was hurrying towards the exit. He'd captured my attention for far longer than I could justify under any other circumstances – I just couldn't take my eyes off him. I'd spent years learning to trust my eyes and knew that if they fixed on something, it was for good reason. And there it was: the answer to why the man who was leaving had caught my attention, was his coat. I'd seen exactly the same one somewhere else. Without even having to think, I knew where: the violent clubber had worn an almost identical one as he'd entered the place earlier on. Could this coat be his? It was a long shot, but some of my colleagues had already felt the full force of the violent clubber's knuckles, and were beginning to tire – I had to see this through.

I raced to the front door and just managed to catch the man before he left. I asked him to make sure that the coat he was wearing was his, and after checking inside it, he confirmed that, although the coat looked like his, it didn't belong to him. The coat was returned to its angry owner, and not a punch more was swung.

Chapter Eleven

INVISIBLE ALLIES

BEING OUT OF YOUR MIND

Only when you are out of your mind can you respond with an appropriate defence. You have to go beyond your mind to react purely to what is. Take, for example, a kick-boxer who is trained to punch and kick his way to safety. He leaves the dojo one night and while on his way home, is attacked. Out come all of his punching and kicking techniques – his mind is programmed to respond in this way. Had he left all his technique behind in the dojo, and walked home with an empty and open mind, he might have spotted the one chance to walk away unhurt: his attacker's face and ears are covered in piercings. A sharp yank of an earring, or piercing anywhere on the body will cause enormous pain, and often profuse bleeding. While the kick-boxer is going at it hell for leather with his programmed response, his one opportunity of escaping unscathed is blown to dust. Not letting your mind call the shots really protects you. It gets you in the moment. Anything less just isn't worth having.

Time is a luxury you don't have when you are under attack – it takes time to think. Get your mind out of the way, and let the rest of you take care of your safety. When serious danger strikes you can either think, or do, but you cannot do both.

You open a kitchen cupboard and a jar falls from the top shelf – notice how you respond. If you catch the jar, you will be operating from a place of no mind. If you think about catching it, you will more than likely end up having to clean up a very messy floor.

I always had zero tolerance when it came to men harassing women in nightclubs. Women have the right to enjoy themselves in peace without having testosterone-filled men breathing down their necks all night long. As far as I was concerned, if a man wasn't able to tell the difference between socializing with a woman, and stalking her, then he was better off somewhere else.

One night I caught a young man hounding a woman on the dance floor. He'd pestered her for a dance for far longer than was socially acceptable, and after two hours of relentlessly nipping at her heels like a hyena stalking a gazelle, he finally wore her down. Out of exasperation, and in a desperate attempt to get him to leave her alone, the woman agreed to a single dance with him.

I kept my eye on the pair for a while. I could see it wouldn't be long before things turned sour – this particular gender tug of war was a pantomime that was only too familiar. My instinct to hang around turned out to be prescient: moments later, the man pushed the woman into a corner, and aggressively tried to coerce her into giving him far more than she'd agreed to. While some bouncers would have left her to fend for herself, for me it was an indiscretion too far. In my book, bullies who made a habit of picking on women were among the worst offenders. Anyway, looking out for the welfare of the most vulnerable clubbers was something I always took seriously. I radioed for backup, caught up with the stranger, and politely asked him to leave. Before I had time to finish what I was saying, the young bully swung for my face.

The next thing I knew, my attacker was face down on the dance floor with me on top of him, pinning him down with both knees and a finger lock. How I ended up in this position is a complete mystery. All I do know is that the punch couldn't have landed because if it had, I would've ended up underneath the young lout, instead of on top of him. When you defend from a place of no mind, you always do whatever needs to be done – and you stay safe doing it.

FLUIDITY

Fluidity is such an important ally to have. When you think about it, life is perpetually on the move and is never still. Having a fluid approach to life gives you the power to keep in step with life's ebbs and flows, so that you are never caught unawares. An attacker strikes without warning – no bother. You gently,

but swiftly deflect the strike and move around him. Things in your day are not
going to plan, but you go with the flow and ride the tide of inconvenience like a
true pro. Before you know it, you have got more done than you had originally
intended.

Some people find change terribly difficult. They are often the sort who only has
one stance on anything. They are also the sort who is unlikely to alter a course
of action once they have committed to it. People who are stiff, and refuse to
bend in life, tend to be the ones who pin all their beliefs on rules. While rules
do have a place, it is vital to keep some fluidity left in the tank. Embracing
fluidity gives you an advantage over others: you never panic because
everything is unfolding just as it should.

*I was once at a private party at a big hall in London. A friend of mine was
having a birthday bash and had invited me along. Although I was there as
a guest, and not as a bouncer, I just couldn't turn off my internal security
switch – a force of habit that turned out to be very useful later on when the
silly hour struck. A couple of hours before the party had fizzled out, a
young man, armed with a broken bottle, charged across the dance floor
towards someone on the other side. Just as he was about to pass me, I
spotted a large bucket of ice on a small table, inches away. There was no
time to think: all I could do was improvise. I grabbed the bucket and threw
all of the ice inside it at the young man's feet. Down he went, slip-sliding
all the way to a stern-looking bouncer who was only too eager to justify
his presence. The dazed young troublemaker was still doing a balletic
glide across the floor, when he was tossed over the bouncer's shoulder like
a butcher's carcass, and carried outside to cool off in the freezing night
air.
Using fluidity to stay safe is classy: it grants you the power to make things
up as you go along. When you live from moment to moment, help can come
dressed as anything – even an ice bucket.*

"I'm gonna punch your f—g lights out! I'm gonna do you some f—g damage, you c—t!" shouted a middle-aged man one night when I refused him entry. I'd decided that the man was definitely better off out than in. He was already abusive enough while sober – what he might be like inside, later on, with a few pints under his belt, didn't bear thinking about. I reasoned that the man's bark was probably worse than his bite – a deliberate tactic to delay any urge to retaliate. I kept quiet, and patiently waited for his outpouring of obscenities to run its course. My silence, though, was an invitation to even more abuse. "You're f—g breaking the law you are! Discriminating bitch! I'll 'ave you! I'm gonna call the police!" he yelled, pointing to a small group of policemen that had been discreetly observing us from the other side of the street. "They'll 'ave you!" he warned, hopping from side to side like a fire-walker on hot coals.

"Be my guest," I replied, with uncharacteristic sangfroid. "Do call them over."

Visibly crushed by my obvious lack of concern, the troublemaker's violent outbursts stopped. He paused for a moment to rethink his strategy: rudeness and threats hadn't succeeded in getting him inside, so perhaps it was time to change tack. With a performance deserving of an Oscar, he turned towards the policemen he knew were watching us, and wailed, "Help! Someone help me! I am the cruel victim of discrimination and am being abused!" He then swallowed enough air to fill an amphitheatre, pointed theatrically in my direction, and bellowed, "I – need – protection – from – HER!"

The troublemaker's pleas were heard. Four no-nonsense policemen immediately raced over to see what all the commotion was about. They took one look at the middle-aged man, came to the conclusion that he was being a thorough nuisance, and carted him off – mid-expletive – to a police van waiting nearby. I could still hear the seething diehard threatening to tear me limb from limb as the van door slammed shut in his face. By all accounts, he screamed blue murder all the way to the police station. The man needed a good hosing down, if you ask me.

MAKING CONNECTIONS

The moon casts an invisible spell from a long way away. It can't be seen or touched. How then, can it have any connection with us? The eternal debate still rages about whether or not our behaviour is influenced by the moon. And yet, all emergency services are stretched to breaking when there is a full moon. As a bouncer, I witnessed much more violence at these times. The slightest magnetic shift even had some people going mad. There is evidence of the moon's power, though many would deny it.

Have a care about dismissing the power of the moon in a hurry. You have nothing to lose, and very likely much to gain from suspending your disbelief. If you live your life without seeing the connections between things, the world becomes a very dangerous place.

A friend of mine was walking down an empty street once, very late at night. She was certain she was being stalked, and in order to find out, she took a sharp turn into another road. The stranger followed her into the same street. My friend is one of those women who really connects with her environment. She believes that, despite outward appearance, there is always something, no matter how obscure, that can help you if you find yourself in trouble. She has no idea how that something might manifest, she just knows that it will. To her, anything within her immediate environment can be a potential ally. As she walked down the empty street where she was being followed, she didn't feel alone. Anything from an empty bottle lying around, to dark spots and shadows, were there to protect her.

My friend could now feel a strong presence behind her: the stranger was only feet away. Terrified, she pulled off one of her boots, and whacked it hard against the bonnet of the nearest car, setting off the alarm. The noise was deafening. Not only did the owner of the car run outside to see what was going on, but several neighbours popped out to have a look-see. My friend was now surrounded with people, and the stalker, not surprisingly, vanished without a trace.

One hot, sultry night at a club in Surrey, management decided to take advantage of the searing heat and turn off all the air conditioning. This would mean that people would flock to the bar and buy more drinks to keep cool, and the club would be the richer for it. The master plan was sound enough, except for one thing: the heat became so unbearable that almost all of the clubbers left. As the bell rang for last orders, only half a dozen people remained, and management was a great deal poorer for it.

Making connections in the world helps you predict possible consequence. It also stops you from looking like a complete wally.

Whenever I was ejecting a woman from a club I always did my homework. Women in clubs are rarely there as a single unit: they're nearly always attached to someone. If you showed a woman to the door you'd often be throwing out one, or more, of the people she was with as well – if she arrived with a male in tow, so much the worse.

One busy night, a young, inexperienced doorman I was working with was asked to throw out a young woman who'd been seen on camera mooning around in a drunken stupor. Before taking a moment to think about how best to get the job done, he leaped into action and, with more eagerness than sense, darted off towards the bar to look for her.

When he found her, she was curled up in a ball sleeping on a chair, with her face in her lap. Always hungry for a war, and only too happy to apply overkill when he found one, my young colleague dived in, clumsily grabbed the limp young woman around the waist, and carelessly dragged her towards the front door. The young woman immediately came to, resisted, and started to scream. My colleague was halfway to the entrance when a man raced up behind him and punched him so hard that he blacked out. The man who attacked my young colleague was the woman's husband. He'd jumped in to protect his wife, understandably.

INNER BALANCE

If you want a balanced life, you must develop inner balance first. Everything comes from your core, your centre. If you try to establish order from the outside, your world might be balanced for a time, but it will not be balanced for long. At the highest level, all separations vanish. There is no such thing as inside and outside – there is only inside. If you haven't found balance there, you won't find it anywhere else.

People who have inner balance are contained. Nothing they do, or say, is extreme. Those who lack it spill out all over the place, in one form or another. Stay away from spillers – they are dangerous.

I'd always feel calm and steady at the beginning of every shift, but an hour or two into the night and I'd usually start to wobble – some heated drama or other would never fail to upset my equilibrium. I'd invariably get drawn into either rescuing someone or restraining them, which would immediately set my inner world out of kilter.

One night I'd had enough of squandering my inner peace and I decided to change. I wanted to see if I was capable of maintaining any semblance of inner balance the next time some crisis erupted. I couldn't help wondering what it would feel like to do that.

I started my first shift at a new venue one night – "lots of regulars" and "lots of trouble", I'd been told. I walked in through the pub doors and was greeted by a somewhat frosty manager. He'd seen so many bouncers come and go. To him, they were all split down the middle and were either cowards or bullies, with nothing in between. I got myself ready and started to patrol the place while I waited for the head doorman to arrive. Tonight, I reminded myself, come hell or high water, I was going to remain inwardly calm. I would see where that led me. I would see if I could do it.

As I passed the main bar, an imposing, grey-haired old man jumped up from his seat, spread his arms wide open, and growled at me like a grizzly. Making a point of taking my time, I pulled out my earpiece and explained to the man that if there was something pressing he wanted to tell me, he'd need to speak up. The old grump laughed out loud, and raised his pint glass as he gave me a supportive wink.

The head doorman turned up soon after and showed me around while introducing me to the realities of the place: it was "rough and unpredictable", and I'd "better watch my back". I was ahead of him. I stuck to my original plan and walked around all night long making sure that nothing, even fear, would tip my inner balance. I stayed out of view when I thought it best, and made my presence felt if the scene warranted it. Whichever way the wind blew, my inner state remained easy.

That night went more smoothly than even the manager could have predicted. At closing time, he waved me over from behind the bar.

"Charly," he beamed, plonking a well earned lager down on the bar in front of me, "it's a rare pleasure to have a trouble-free night. I love your balanced approach. Are you staying with us?"

That night gave me my first taste of what inner balance felt like. It showed me how a more temperate way of being can influence the world around you. I did stay at that pub for another ten months and in all that time, the only thing to be so much as thrown, was the odd angry stare.

INTENT

A powerful intention, coupled with an immediate follow-through, will give you formidable results. You are most likely to achieve your goal when there is no gap between the intention you hold, and the physical execution of it. If you ever find yourself wanting to achieve the seemingly impossible, hold that thought as strongly as you can until you carry out your intention – see where that takes you.

You don't always have to act out an intention physically to stay safe. Often, just holding a strong sense of intent within is enough. A street predator who is on the lookout for someone to pounce on, is scanning for someone who dithers; someone who is clueless about where they are off to, and what they will do when they get there. You come along, and it is clear from the way you walk, from your expression, and from your energy, that you know exactly who is who, and what is what. On the basis that all street thugs need an easy life – time is not on their side – they won't bother to attack you if you are solid and have a strong sense of self. They would only end up having to work twice as hard, and twice as long. Never undervalue the power of intent – your average street thug doesn't.

I had a real opportunity of seeing just what kind of stuff I was made of one night when I found myself having to stop a hugely obese man, who'd passed out from alcohol poisoning, from crashing to the floor. In a moment of drunken exuberance he'd upset several crates of empty glasses

that had been on the stage above him, and was only seconds from landing on a bed of glass. I'd seen people bellyflop onto glass before and knew how bloody it could be. An eleven stone body landing on a glass-covered floor was bad enough, but a person weighing well over twenty stone might not survive the experience. In any event, a mop up operation was the last thing I needed.

The intoxicated clubber was now about to plummet to the floor and certain injury. I pushed my ten and a half stone mass into his body, and pinned him against the wall. Now that I had him almost vertical, I knew I could cope for a couple of minutes – I'd radioed for help. Things, though, quickly took a turn for the worse. "Charly!" came the response from the head doorman, "I can't help at the moment – a major problem outside!" In my entire career as a bouncer I had never come so close to giving up. I was now out of breath, and my arms were burning from the strain of having to hold up the over twenty-stoner – I was a hair's breadth from letting the Almighty sort it all out.

Then, a flashback – a vivid memory of how only two years before I'd gone for my first black belt. I'd had to smash through four tiles with my fist in order to get it. If I failed after two goes, I wouldn't get my belt. I did fail – twice. The experience stung because that day I'd seen women half as strong as me succeed. They'd intended to smash through the tiles so completely, that they did. My power of intent that day had been lacking, and I knew it. I went for my black belt again some months later and this time I blasted through the tiles without even drawing blood. I was capable of directing my will after all. Could I reconnect with it now?

The over twenty-stoner's head and shoulders were now beginning to drop again. I quickly wedged my lower arm under his chin, and flipped his head back. As the weight of his upper body fell back, so did the rest of him. I grabbed his belt and, with all the force of a ram charging at a brick wall, pushed his body against the stage to straighten him up. To make sure he stayed up, I edged my feet further out to give me more pushing power, and dug in with everything. Just as my knees were about to buckle, two of my colleagues arrived to carry the over twenty-stoner to safety. Against insurmountable odds, and with nothing more than the power of my intent to see me through, I'd kept the heavyweight from crashing to the floor for over ten minutes.

BEING A SPIRITUAL BOUNCER

Words can be dangerous. A harsh word can cause offence, and if left to fester, can cause disease. When you allow dark energy in, it is vital to get rid of it quickly. There are all kinds of ways that you can do this. One way to spiritually bounce out the toxic imprint left from hostile, angry words, is to mentally stick it in an envelope, and immediately mark it "return to sender". As you do this, take a few moments to really see it happening: the more intensely you visualize toxic energy leaving you, the more effectively it will travel back to source. Another way to rid yourself of someone else's energetic garbage, is to imagine a large cancel button, right in the middle of your forehead, that blitzes every verbal unpleasantness as it hits you.

My favourite way to spiritually bounce out other people's energetic waste, is to give it to Mother Earth. Mother Earth is a powerful alchemist: she will clean any kind of energy, no matter how dark. If someone projects anger towards you, and you feel that anger all through your body, imagine it gathering in a tight ball somewhere in your body – your solar plexus, for example. Hold it there, then go outside to Mother Earth. When you have reached a spot where you feel strongly connected to her, pull all that energetic rubbish out of your solar plexus with your hands. Keep going until you feel there is no more left. As you pull, try and picture the dark energy leaving you. Try and get a clear sense of what that toxic energy looks like. Is it a colour? Is it alive? Does it remind you of an animal? Is the energy shaped like invisible tendrils, or is it more like an amorphous, cloudy mass? As soon as you feel that you have removed all the unwanted energy, just stand for a moment holding it in your hands. When you are ready, kneel down and tenderly ask Mother Earth to take it from you. Say, "Great Mother, I humbly ask you to take this energy from me because it no longer serves me. I love you and thank you." Then gently lay the palms of your hands on the earth, and feel all the unwanted energy flowing into her.

Violent words are poison. They contaminate everything they touch. So whatever crud makes its way in, make sure you spiritually bounce it out straight away – don't hang around. If someone came around and dumped a truckload of manure on your immaculate, green lawn, I suspect you would jump to get rid of it. Why would you do any less for yourself?

Real spiritual bouncers were so rare on the doors that they stuck out like sore thumbs. Whenever I did spot one I'd always try and work closely with them – if I could. They were always a delight to work with because they

were so flexible when it came to letting everything drop – they didn't dwell on things. They'd quickly dispose of whatever verbal garbage didn't belong to them, and move on. Unfortunately, a friend of mine I worked with briefly on the doors wasn't able to do this. He used to get terribly upset by some of the foul language that clubbers would throw at him. He'd seethe and breathe hellfire for an entire night whenever someone abused him verbally. He'd hold onto all the dirty linen for an age. The problem was that when he had to concentrate on doing his job, he just couldn't. One night he was so indignant about a man who'd sworn at him two nights before that he accidentally allowed an underager into the club. The head doorman fired him on the spot.

I refused a verbally abusive man entry one night: I could smell alcohol off his breath, and told him as much. He argued that his friends were inside the club and that if I didn't let him in, one of them would come out to the front door and "punch my lights out". I didn't like being threatened, but instead of giving the man the verbal dusting down that I felt he deserved, I held back. This, I reasoned, was an ideal opportunity to see what could be achieved by spiritually bouncing back all the man's darkness to him.

I took a split second to imagine myself holding up a mirror, and I visualized all of his verbal rubbish being reflected back to him – like a laser beam. Actually, I pictured it going back to him tenfold. Doing this served me well because as soon as I'd got rid of all the man's energetic negativity, I was clean. With balance restored, I was prepared for whatever came next.

The drunkard's threat, as it turned out, hadn't been an idle one. With my back turned, one of his cronies rushed up behind me from inside, and tried to push me out of the way so that his friend could get in. Because I wasn't holding any resentment from earlier on, I was able to concentrate on what was happening around me, so I saw him coming. As he reached for me, I dropped to his feet, and watched him fall head over heels all the way out to the pavement, where he landed next to his friend with a splat. Not carrying other people's negative baggage makes you so much quicker off the mark.

LEARNING TO SEE WITH YOUR FEELINGS

Not judging by outward appearance is vital where your safety is concerned. Your eyes can deceive you – not all street thugs look like down-and-outs. When you are out and about, learn to see with your feelings, not just your eyes. When you start using your feelings to look out at the world, you will find yourself energetically matching the person you are looking at. You will begin to mirror what they are feeling – this gives you power. Get some practice in and start by trying to gauge the feelings of those close to you. It is much easier to get precious feedback on whether you have been accurate from the people you know. Then head out to your local High Street and see if you can sense what people are feeling there. Gently reach out to them from your heart, as that will open up the connection between you more.

Everyone has the ability to sense the feelings of others. People have always had this gift, but few ever use it. Most people have forgotten that it is even there. Developing the ability to see with your feelings is a defence staple worth having, because as soon as you are no longer judging a book by its cover, you are seeing things as they really are. Only relying on externals as a way of staying safe is overrated, and dangerous – violent men wear pinstriped suits, as well as bomber jackets. So focus on the subtle; focus on what is going on with people inwardly. The surface of the sea might look safe enough, but does that mean it all is?

Although searching clubbers as they entered was arguably a bouncer's most important job, I always made a point of taking as many precautions as I could at the front door, to minimize any likelihood for trouble inside later on. A colleague of mine searched a man one night and, satisfied that he wasn't concealing anything he shouldn't have been, gave him the thumbs up. Just as the man started heading for the dance floor, I waved him back and suggested to my colleague that he frisk him again. This time, he did so a little more thoroughly and found a knife hidden beneath the man's trouser leg, tucked into his sock. My colleague was clearly spooked. "How did you do that Charly? You got X-ray vision or somethin'?" he asked, taking a step back while deciding what to make of me. I assured him that seeing through walls and people's trousers wasn't a talent I possessed, but that I'd become suspicious of the man as soon as he'd entered. "He seemed a bit too eager to cooperate," I remarked, being more

than a little economical with the truth. "Looked as if he had something to hide."

That was the abridged version. The full version contained a good deal more to set alarm bells ringing. While I'd been closely watching the man being searched the first time, I'd tuned into him so completely that I began to feel exactly what he was feeling. You can often tell when you're picking up on the feelings of others because your mood changes – suddenly. If your inner state does a pendulum swing, and goes from calm to chaotic in under a second, then someone physically close by often has something to do with it. As I stood watching the man being searched, my inner tranquillity evaporated and was replaced by mounting tension. Fear gripped my chest like a ton weight, and I became breathless. I knew that these feelings didn't belong to me. The man being searched saw me studying him and quickly guessed that he'd become transparent. Realizing I was on to him, he forced an uncomfortable friendliness, and used it as a veneer to mask all outward sign of his growing trepidation. But I wasn't watching him physically: I was watching him inwardly. I was using my feelings as a bridge to see all of his. And if I could see his fear, then I could also see his reason for having it. As the man had made his way to the bar after being searched, I tapped my colleague on the shoulder and explained that, perhaps, things were not quite as they appeared.

I spent years on the doors searching people, not only with my eyes, but with my feelings. People are what they feel – not what they think. If you can become a mirror and reflect what people are feeling, you will get to see them as they really are. That night, I honoured my feelings and went with them. For my colleagues, this was the flimsiest of evidence to go on. For me, it was always enough.

Chapter Twelve

THE DOOR OPENS

THE ULTIMATE BATTLE

Mastering the self is the ultimate battle. It is known as the ultimate battle because it is the toughest – the tests and challenges you face there cannot be equalled. It is waged on the invisible plain, and is the only true measure of power. When the battle has been won, there is nothing more to prove, and there is nowhere to go. You have set your spirit free, and the world no longer defines you.

The ultimate battle is not for the faint-hearted. Spend a day not having a single negative thought. Easy, isn't it?

When you have been waging war to conquer the inner self for long enough, and won, you will find yourself in a place where things just are as they are. This is because you have learnt not to judge yourself. When you no longer judge yourself, you no longer judge anyone else. When you have done judging everything, you will have no more arguments with the world, and the world will therefore have none with you. The ultimate battle is, after all, the final battle.

A man approached the front door who I recognized as one of our most hardened alcoholics. Most nights he'd arrive sober, and once inside would prop up the bar and down as much alcohol as his wiry frame would allow. We'd sometimes be harsh with him – and brutal. Well before half-time he'd be grabbed, shoved out through the front door, and insulted for being

the drunk that he was. Tonight, though, he was already over the limit before he'd even reached the bar. His breath reeked of alcohol and his legs could barely keep him upright. He stood in the doorway, goggle-eyed and docile, anxiously waiting to see if I'd let him in.

For some unfathomable reason, his lack of sobriety wasn't a major concern that night. It was as if something had snapped within me. Normally, I would have turned him away without blinking. The man had, after all, made my life impossible the previous week when, as a result of yet another of his alcoholic binges, he'd collapsed in the men's loo. I spent forty minutes trying to unlock the toilet door and when I finally got him out, I told him not to come back – ever.

While I stood in the doorway deciding whether or not to let the man through, I felt as if I were seeing with different eyes. As if it were the most natural thing in the world, I warmly ushered the man in. Not believing his luck, he shook my hand until I thought it would drop off, and raced to the bar with the speed of a jackrabbit.

Life was never quite the same after that. There was just no need to judge anymore. If people wanted to self-destruct, then that was their business. I made it my business to have compassion for all forms of human compulsion and frailty, and from then on, all were welcomed in through the doors – within reason.

Late that night when I was alone, I wandered outside to take a moment to acknowledge the enormity of the step I'd taken in no longer judging the world. All I had for company was an empty street and a starlit sky that seemed to belong only to me – the hallowed watchers of my emerging awareness. With eyes closed, and grinning from ear to ear, I lifted my face to the stars and quietly gave thanks. I knew I was free because what people did simply didn't matter anymore. The world was just perfect as it was.

BEING INWARDLY DIRECTED

In the world of quantum physics, it is now generally accepted that the outcome of an event can be influenced by the fact that you are observing it. This isn't news to the female warrior who spends her life shaping outer circumstances from within. She knows that she is able to affect the world of form merely by being conscious of it.

When you take your lead from within to create a result in the world, you are inwardly directed. You could also say that you are living inside out.

The female warrior uses her own inner promptings to stay safe. She knows that looking to others for answers is risky – hearsay is often unreliable, and can be easily distorted. So she cuts a path through life on her own, and tunes into her subtle feelings and intuitions to avoid danger. If there is any tension brewing in a crowd, she will feel it early enough to be miles away by the time danger strikes. If you were to ask a female warrior what she would do if attacked, she would say, "I wouldn't be there."

A colleague of mine and I were given an assignment: we both had to spend the night tracking the movements of a man who was a known drug dealer. The manager wanted to try and catch him red-handed while doing his worst. Although this wouldn't be easy because the nightclub we were working at was vast – eight dance floors and as many bars to keep an eye on – it was one of those jobs that I took on with relish as it gave me another opportunity to fine-tune my more subtle skills.

My colleague and I split up, and while I managed to keep tabs on the man until the wee hours, my colleague made a complete hash of things. Whenever the head doorman pressed him on the whereabouts of the man he was supposed to be shadowing, he was clueless. After having spent the better part of two hours losing sight of his target, he was asked to step down and let me handle the tracking – much to his annoyance.

Although my colleague and I both had the same job to do, and the same level of experience to do it, there was a major difference in our strategies: while he acted only on information coming to him from those around him, I didn't. I trusted that my own inner cues would lead me to the man: a hunch, a gut feeling, even an image in my mind would be enough to enable me to find him. I also pictured myself as him: what would I do, and where would I move to, if I were him? Keeping my inner radar tuned meant that no matter where, or how far away the drug dealer was, I always had a direct line to him.

Just as the bell rang for last orders, our drug dealer started doing some trade right under my nose. My being a witness to his subterfuge turned out to be his undoing, and after many more successful trackings at that particular nightspot, I became respectfully known as "The Tail".

THE POWER IN SOFTNESS

Softness is a portal; it is a doorway to power that will only open if you are knocking gently. The power that lies beyond softness resonates at a particular frequency and if you are not resonating in sympathy with it, you won't be allowed through because you won't be recognized. There is an infinite number of routes to softening – as many as there are people. It was exhaustion that led me there. On one of the most challenging nights I can recall, I had spent so long trying to physically restrain one drunken lout after another, that I had reached a state of near physical and mental collapse. I was so tired that I couldn't even argue. Exhaustion proved a most trusted friend that night because it denied me the energy to make war. With war out of the picture, I could be lovingly guided towards something I had never considered. It was also the only avenue left: softness.

To soften, you must become like ice that melts into water. When you start to thaw from the hard, icy state that has become familiar, and you begin to change into a less dense form, the softening process has begun. At this point, your resistance to change will have started to lessen, and you might feel vulnerable and naked. With resistance, something else begins to die: any desire for control. Not forcing things will feel like a giant leap in the dark; it will feel as if you have taken your foot off the gas pedal and allowed something else to keep the car going.

Softening is a kind of test: only once you have demonstrated your ability to surrender to something you can't see, will the power that lies beyond softness let you through. The biblical reference to the meek inheriting the earth is an example of how true power only comes to those who hold an inner softness. Once you have become like water, you must go deeper into softness. To be welcomed in through the doorway you must become water that has evaporated into mist. When you are weightless and free enough to become pure essence and spirit, the power on the other side of softness will claim you as its own. It is this frequency that it has been waiting for. It is your lightness of being that is the key that can open the door.

The power that lies beyond softness will know the second you have gone from water to mist, for you will have become softness itself in body, mind, and spirit. Once every aspect of you is bathed in softness, you are ready to receive true power because only now are you congruent with it. You understand that you are not the origin of power, but merely the vessel that can hold it.

If you can suspend your disbelief in a higher power for just a moment, and open to softness a little, you might be given a sneak preview of what lies beyond it. Softness is a window to power, and if you dare to peek through it, you might decide that you prefer the view. You might even decide to go through it and stay on the other side for good. We have a sacred contract to tread softly as we walk. Softness opens all channels to a divine power that has a way of making everything come out right.

If you want to physically move someone you can do it in two ways: you can either use physical force, or you can apply softness through your voice, demeanour, and presence. Physically grappling with someone to get them to move might look impressive, but controlling someone bodily, without even touching them, is far more powerful – you have used the least, to achieve the most.

A drunken woman had somehow managed to clamber onto one of the bars and was making life impossible for the barmen. The manager of the nightclub was worried that the barmen might decide to take matters into their own hands – legally, a woman is only allowed to be physically handled by a female bouncer. If any of the barmen had dealt with things on their own, and put a foot wrong, the woman would have been well within her rights to sue the nightclub. The manager was always at his most offensive when under pressure, and this was a delicate situation requiring an approach that was quite beyond his scope. "Charly! Pull that f—g woman off the upstairs bar! I don't f—g care how you do it, just get her off. Now!"

I shot upstairs to the room where all this was going on and when I got there, my heart sank. The only way I could get to the bar was to cut through a sea of clubbers packed so tightly, you couldn't have squeezed a slice of lemon in between them. I had to find a way through: the manager was one of the most vile I'd ever known – and that was without a lawsuit. I braced myself for the crowd, and pushed in.

I managed to get halfway across the floor when a man jumped in front of me, blocking my only path to the bar. Chatting away with his back turned, he had no idea that I was there, and even less idea that he was blocking my way. I shouted to get his attention, but the pounding of the speakers close by drowned me out. I tried giving him a firm prod with my radio antenna, but what with so many clubbers all shunting him from pillar to post, my extra poke didn't make any difference.

I stood on the tips of my toes and peered over the mass of heads all bobbing up and down, to check things at the bar. The woman was now doing an ungainly catwalk stagger up and down the length of the bar, and the head barman looked as if he was about to lose his usual composure. With only half the length of the floor left between me and the bar, I was so close to being able to sort all this out, and yet still so far. Surrounded by a moist blanket of flickering, multicoloured silhouettes all rising and falling to a single beat, I imagined myself a solitary minnow lost in a whirring school of fish. I'd always felt uncomfortable in the middle of crowds, and as a bouncer had always been on the outside of any crowd, looking in. Now finding myself stuck in the middle of one, unable to look out, was fast becoming a most unwelcome exercise in trust. The crowd, oblivious, and growing increasingly indifferent to my need for space, began to close in. Vulnerable and unable to move, I stood absolutely still, closed my eyes, and went within. In my mind's eye, I soared high above sounds, lights, and motion, and found myself looking down. I was a raptor hovering over prey, and could now see myself in context: below was a circle, a dancing carnival of shadows all spinning around a central axis. I was this axis. I was the hub that kept the carnival turning. I was the part that didn't move, so that every other part could. I opened my eyes and brought what I'd seen above, down to earth. My stillness, now set against this most phantasmagorical of backdrops, was more intense than ever. And in that contrast lay my answer: a drop of softness in an ocean of turmoil was all I needed to clear the path. I brushed the man blocking my way lightly with the back of my fingers, then gently slid them over his arm like a feather. He jumped out of his skin, I'd got his attention, and the rest was a walk in the park.

A young, inexperienced colleague and I decided one night to toss a coin for the next job. The nightclub was so quiet that there wasn't enough work to go around. No sooner had I won the toss, than a bad-tempered bar manager started screaming for some help from security. "Charly! Sling out the bloke sitting near the bar! He's drinking us dry!"

My young colleague had already tried unsuccessfully to get the man to leave earlier on, and was somewhat crestfallen that I'd been called in to get the job done. He became defensive and didn't hide the fact that, in his opinion, if a man couldn't sort something out, a woman had no chance. I pointed out to him that there was an alternative to using force: softness, I explained, was often a much more powerful way to control behaviour. I put it to him that I'd be able to get the troublemaker to leave without even touching him – and maintain a gentle demeanour while doing it. "Watch and learn," I advised, tapping my nose.

When we caught up with the obstreperous clubber, he was embroiled in a heated verbal slurring match with one of his beer buddies. "Good evening, sir," I said, playfully snatching his attention. "I think you've probably had quite enough. I would be most grateful if you would finish your drink and make your way out with me."

Both men slammed down their pint glasses – not so hard as to spill any of their precious Newcastle Brown finest – and expressed outrage at having been so rudely interrupted. "I'm busy! Can't you see I'm having an intellectual discussion with my mate?" spluttered the man I was hoping to escort out. "Do your worst! I'm not moving an inch!"

Radiating a quiet confidence, I suggested to the man, who had now turned around to continue arguing with his beer buddy, that he might be a little more alcoholically challenged than he realized. "If you can show me how sober you are by standing up," I said, deliberately placing myself between him and his drinking partner, "you might not need to come with me to the door after all."

In order to be rid of me, and to save himself from further pestering, the man complied. He gripped the arms of his chair to steady himself, and with great effort slowly heaved himself up. "There you are, see!" he shouted, spraying me with beer. "Pool cue straight! Now p—s off!"

Satisfied that he'd convinced me of his sobriety, he went to plonk himself back down in his chair but missed the target. Had it not been for the surprisingly quick reactions of his inebriated beer buddy helping him to his seat, he would have landed on the floor bottom first. I watched the whole palaver and struggled to conceal a smile.

Once the troublemaker was safely reinstalled in his chair, I softly coaxed him a little more.

"I'm sure you can do much better than that. If you really want to show me how sober you are, why don't you give yourself a real challenge and walk over to the bar?"

The man's shaky legs not only carried him all the way to the bar, but all the way out to the front door as well. He staggered right past the bouncers outside and just kept going. I used this tactic a lot on the doors. Sometimes people would fall for it, and sometimes they wouldn't. It was a peach, though, when it worked. People will do almost anything to prove you wrong.

Chapter Thirteen

END RUN

SELF-WORTH

If you don't have much self-worth, chances are your personal safety won't be a priority. When you scratch the surface of women in violent relationships, you always come up with the same fact: they have low self-esteem. A woman who leaves her safety unchecked is entering into an unloving contract with herself. Many women say that being in an abusive relationship is just plain bad luck. I say we all choose what comes into our lives. The choices we make always match our measure of self-worth.

A powerful exercise to do to get the measure of your self-worth, is to place one coin of every denomination in a row in front of you – do the same with notes. You now have one long row of coins and notes ranging from a one penny piece, to a fifty pound note. With a completely open and honest heart, look at each one, and when you are ready, pick up the one that you feel matches your self-worth. Hold it to your heart, and say to yourself, "I am worth —" On a fairly regular basis, do this exercise again to see if there has been a shift. As you start to move up the monetary scale, compare your results with the choices you are making of late. As you plot the chart of your soaring self-esteem, you might begin to notice that you are starting to attract those with the same level of self-worth. As you continue spiralling ever upwards towards a deeper, inward sense of worthiness, dark energies won't be able to cling on, and your old world, with all its violence and chaos, will start to fall away. Eventually, you will have become a fifty pound note, and you will find yourself in a place where you get to be the most you can possibly be. When you arrive there, you will turn and look at the distance you have covered, and you will laugh and wonder why it took you so long to see the obvious: that there is more danger lurking in a penny, than in a fifty pound note.

Stag parties were something to behold. One night a young man decided to drink himself to oblivion two days before his wedding. He stood at the bar the whole night and downed so much beer that he'd have been much better off ordering by the trough. With his friends egging him on, and in order to impress some women standing nearby, he went at it like a young buck let loose in a field of deer. The man's thirst for oblivion seemed more like a death wish than a celebration of things to come.

I could see he was close to keeling over, so I stood in a dark corner and quietly observed things from close by. Just as the groom-to-be was about to knock back one pint too many, I got ready for his inevitable drop to the floor. I'd had my fill of scraping the alcoholically undisciplined off of nightclub floors and to make life easier, would always try to catch them before they toppled over. I walked up to the young buck, who was now so drunk that he couldn't line up his glass with his mouth, and politely asked him to accompany me to the exit to have a chat. Doddery, and swaying like a marionette, he swung round and told me that if I didn't leave him alone, I'd be wearing the beer he was drinking.

And that was the straw that broke the camel's back. I knew then, without a shadow of a doubt, that I'd reached the end of the line. Getting sworn at, punched, and covered in lager on a fairly regular basis just didn't seem appropriate anymore. I felt worthy of better company.

As soon as closing time came, I headed straight for the manager's office to tell him that I wouldn't be back. "Which other club you going to, Charly?" he asked, worried that one of his best bouncers had been poached by a rival club.

"None," I replied, handing him back my radio for the last time. "I'm jacking in my job as a bouncer. No more door work for me." That moment was sweet. The thought of finding something else to do that reflected my self-worth was even sweeter.

DETACHMENT

Should you decide to have a stab at getting a sense of what detachment feels like, spend a day repeating to yourself, "I am here in the world as a spectator, not as a participant." When you finally understand that you aren't here to get involved, you no longer feel obliged to join in, and you disengage. When this happens, you are no longer emotionally plugged in to the world. The world will register this, and when it does, you become invisible. You literally slip underneath its radar, and danger won't stalk you as it can't see you.

Imagining yourself as a female turtle is a good way to get into the spirit of detachment. One species of female turtle can swim three thousand miles in a year – one of the longest journeys any animal can make. You can imagine that she encounters many perils as she travels, but she slowly and gracefully swims the ocean as if in her own world – as if she is apart. Other creatures might notice her serenely pass by, but surprisingly, she isn't often considered as lunch. It is as if she is in the sea, but not of it. There is great safety in detachment. When you silently coast on the periphery of life, you become an outsider. If you are going to give your average shark the slip, I don't know of a better way to do it.

Being detached also means that you are putting distance between you and life. The more you move away from the mainstream, the less likely you are to be taken in with people's nincompooperies and mindless acts of violence. When you become detached, it feels as if you are on top of a high mountain. From that height, you are able to get a much clearer picture of what goes on beneath. Like the eagle that soars high above ground, you have the advantage of foresight. Detachment is about living above life, rather than beneath it. The next time you feel that life is getting on top of you, head for the hills.

I was patrolling the lobby of a busy nightclub one night, when I saw two young men giving each other a verbal pasting. I charged in and, against my better judgement, got involved in their bickering. The two men in question were having a lovers' tiff, and I found myself doing something foolish: I took sides. I got emotionally involved and decided that one of the men was bullying the other. I gently tried to separate them in order to escort the bully of the piece to the door, but the second I touched him, the other one swung for me and tried to drag me to the floor. That's the crash course in learning about how to become detached.

WALKING AWAY

It is no defeat to walk away from verbal abuse. Walking away is a sign of maturity. It shows that you are not operating from base level, and are wise enough to know that no good can ever come from engaging with negative energy. It also shows that you are taking responsibility for the well-being of those close to you by making your own safety a priority – no person is an island.

The dynamics of walking away are something to be aware of. If someone swears at you, consider the possibility that the foul language isn't coming from them. Consider that they are just the vehicle through which it is being communicated. Foul energy manifests through people's words and is generated from an invisible, malevolent place. The dark side delights in trying to pull the easily converted over to its side, so treat all verbal abuse as a test. If someone disrespects you with words, just walk away. You win on two counts when you do: you stay safe, and you live to give the dark side its marching orders another day.

The next time you find yourself indulging in a bit of verbal sparring, notice how your solar plexus feels – that is where your anger is held. Whatever fire you are using to win an argument comes from there. What happens with that fire you are putting out is interesting: when you verbally try to clobber an opponent, you become energetically attached to them. The angry words that you are sending out act like glue, and you end up getting stuck to the person you are trying to demolish. A good way to see this is to think of invisible tendrils projecting out from your solar plexus, and hooking onto your sparring partner as you speak – or shout. Your opponent is going through the same process: their anger is projecting invisible tendrils that are trying to attach to you. In no time, you are both energetically connected to each other, and the channels are open for things to get worse.

Locking horns with anyone is quite an intimate thing to do. When you attach to another person, for any reason, you are entering into a relationship with them. Before your next slanging match, take a second to ask yourself if it is a relationship you want with the person you are about to lay into, or distance.

It took me years to learn how to walk away from arguments – I always had to have the last word. Eventually, I began to see that doing things this way just made me feel bad. I decided I didn't enjoy being consumed with hellfire anymore, and anyway, I'd outgrown it – one night I had a chance to find out just how much. A man walked in through the front door and asked me some very personal questions that I had no intention of answering. When I refused to satisfy his curiosity, he took offence and let rip: he boiled, and spat, and hissed – a real pressure cooker about to blow. I'd never come across a more disproportionate reaction. All I'd said to him was "no". I calmly focussed on any fluttering in my midsection, and waited. Incredibly, there was no anger there, and no desire to hit back. For once, I didn't feel the need to lash out.

As I turned to walk away, the man erupted. Incandescent with rage that I'd refused to play ball, he glared at me as if I'd physically punched him. All the unexpressed emotional fire that he'd projected towards me hadn't managed to find a target, and like a coiled spring had shot straight back to him and thumped him in the stomach.

Dishing the dirt isn't all it's cracked up to be. When you mud-sling, you not only squander precious energy, you also get back whatever filth you sent out. Walking away is an act of power. It's also the cleaner option.

GOODBYE DRAMA

Drama is a magnificent distraction. You become so focussed on whatever carry-on is taking place, that you become a sitting duck. Being a sitting duck in a public place can present you with some dicey prospects where your safety is concerned. You walk down a street alone at night while having a row with your boyfriend on your mobile, and are so absorbed with the argument you are having, that you don't see the street thug rushing you from behind. You might say that drama "just happens", and that there is no way to see an attack coming. If this really is how you see things, then drama has you. And it always will have you until you understand that there are always signals alerting you to trouble ahead. Drama is in place to stop you noticing them – its job is to keep you blinkered.

Next Christmas, give yourself the best present you have ever had and drop drama in the toilet where it belongs.

Drama is the situation, and struggle is how you get there. The more you struggle, the more drama you will have. If you like, struggle is the petrol that fuels all the drama. Having a drama-filled life steers you away from your centre. You become a ship without an anchor, and you find yourself being pulled along with any prevailing tide. This may be the way you want to be pulled, or it may not: the point is, you are pulled anyway. As you get dragged along to who knows where, you will whine and moan about your lot. You will struggle to blazes because you have completely forgotten that you have, on some level, agreed to be dragged. You will be in good company, though: other strugglers will be with you, which is just as well as it will guarantee lots more drama.

The key that unlocks all of this mayhem is to refuse to play the role of victim. You just decide that you want to play another role instead, and you jump ship. You hurl yourself off the drama merry-go-round, and cut the ties that were binding you to perpetual struggle. The moment you do, you are no longer a struggler. And with no more struggle left in the tank to fuel any more drama, you are free.

Your new found freedom might feel scary at first, and your life might seem terrifyingly empty – a huge void exists where drama used to be. But take heart, because the real fun is just about to begin. That void is your only true source of power. It is the only merry-go-round of any interest to the female warrior.

The world would have you believe that life must be full to bursting with drama. The world is telling you this because it wants you to get hooked on it. Drama can slip into your life quietly at first, but be careful that it doesn't end up controlling it. Watch carefully for the earliest signs of it, and stamp it out like you would a bug – indulging in drama is an addiction. Going cold turkey and giving it up is hard, but think about it: you lose enormous amounts of energy and give your power away every time you get caught up in some drama or other.

Study the lives of those who are drama-free: life for them seems balanced and easy. They seem to glide through their day, rather than battle their way through it. If some obstacle does happen to fall into their path, they are quite happy just going around it; or under it; or over it. The thing is, they don't get out a sledge hammer and try to bludgeon their way through it.

Living like this leaves them with plenty of energy to invest in their personal safety. By the time an attacker strikes, they are up the road having coffee and muffins in Starbucks.

A nightclub is any drama addict's paradise. As I patrolled the dance floors of London and beyond, I felt as if I were watching the world in microcosm: addictions to alcohol, drugs, sex, money, power, and drama, all collected in one small space. I often used to joke to some of my colleagues that I felt a bit like a parent at a toddler's ice cream and jelly party – the reality was very different. I was keenly aware that I was witness to the collective human shadow; the unconscious, hidden part which only surfaces when the conscious mind is dulled. Alcohol and drugs are the perfect tools to reduce the conscious mind to mush and open gateways for mass hidden demons. I was there not so much to stem the flow of physical violence: I was mostly there to constantly massage, and coax, the collective human shadow into submission – if I could. Many people, who seemed affable enough on entering, would turn into bullies and sadists soon after walking in. Often, whole groups of people would arrive straight from the office. They saw a nightclub as a sort of emotional trash can where everything unconsciously pathological within them could be dumped. When I first started working on the doors all this excited me; drama excited me – that's why I signed up for it. But one night, cracking the whip as ringmaster to force every kind of human unconscious monstrosity back into its cage had worn thin, and drama no longer seemed cool.

For a while, there was a gap; an uncomfortable, empty hole where drama had been. I was in that twilight zone where the old no longer applies, but the new has yet to appear. A faint, emergent presence slowly moved in to act as a substitute. It obscured drama just long enough for me to consider a new possibility: could I get as much done – if not more – by doing less? And then it happened. One brutal, bloody night, softness sneaked in when my guard was down. I was so worn out that before I'd even found the strength to bounce her out, she had already weaved her magic.

Softness was like a new toy at first. I was a child playing with something that I couldn't possibly understand. Later on, I discovered that the power in softness wasn't a toy at all, but a force; an energy that connects every single thing that humans can conceive of, and then transcends it. And here, right here in the damp, half-lit, spirit decaying world of club land was where the heart of softness had been beating all along. Here in the half-life, softness had lovingly spread her wings so wide, that every evil imaginable could thrive, unjudged. Invisible and infinite, she had waited patiently just beyond the dark to be of service to those who could bear a most powerful reality. I had dared to reach beyond the tawdry, somnambulant world of human illusion. I had tasted the emptiness of the half-life and yearned for a kinder place.

I had come of age. I was no longer a child playing with something beyond my comprehension because I could now behold the power in softness without needing to run. I'd found the strength to withstand the glare of her beauty from something she'd promised: that as long as I walked in softness, I would be so much bigger than anything else. Most of all, I would have no limits.

My belief that inside and outside were separate could no longer hold. Softness was the best of foils to teach me that one was merely an extension of the other. Each time I plopped a drop of softness into a violent situation, the effect would be instant, and powerful. I grew to delight in the ease with which the harsh would be overpowered by the soft. I grew to respect it so much, that I took softness within and used her wonder to soothe my infernal chatter. Softness, like a doting Mother, quickly set about healing and transmuting my unseen darkness, and without so much as a whimper most of my destructive habits vanished. Like a silken veil, softness had floated so deeply into my being that she had become my only point of reference.

Life became effortless after that. I found myself patrolling the dance floors of club land with the gentleness of a summer breeze. Whatever problem needed fixing, I'd turn to softness. A furious clubber would have nothing to fight against; an arrogant bouncer would be humbled. A few weeks before my last night on the doors, a fellow bouncer accused me of being soft in the head. The worst thing you could ever level at a bouncer was the word "soft". I was flattered: softness had already become my new cool.

I spent my last nights on the doors as if in a dream. Like a person a short time before death, I was straddling two different worlds – the body remained, but the spirit had flown. I'd found a way out of the human realm of make-believe, and before I'd even noticed, my old world had quietly slipped away. As I walked out through the doors on my final shift, I turned for a last time to gaze at all the insanity I was leaving behind. I smiled, lifted my hand to my lips, and blew it all softly away with a kiss. With a fresh wind on my back, and a chorus of birdsong beckoning me home, I left. How I'd get home was anybody's guess. But I'd travel with a soft heart, and a light step. Yes. That would be my way there.

AFTERWORD

You are not a medicine woman because of what you do, or because of what technique you use to heal. Neither are you a medicine woman because of what you have studied, with whom, or for how long. The only real measure a medicine woman has to judge her worth as a holder of sacred space, lies with who "*she*" is.

A true medicine woman understands that the tools of her trade cannot define the power of her medicine. She gauges the effectiveness of her medicine from her own inner landscape: is there humility enough inside her to connect to a power she recognizes as so much greater than herself? Is there a compassion for humankind so vast, that she can detach from the world out of a love that can no longer carry judgement?

If these gifts live within you, then you must already have cultured softness – if you have inner softness, you have everything else. When you take care of softness, everything else takes care of itself. That is a medicine woman's yardstick.

Using her softness, the medicine woman draws an invisible circle in the air and sets your spirit free. Where does your spirit fly to? Through softness, the medicine woman gently sweeps you to infinity; to the now. All true healing takes place there, or not at all.

ABOUT THE AUTHOR

Charly Flower trained as a classical singer at Trinity College of Music in London. She then went on to train as a journalist at the London College of Printing, and it was during this time that she began her training as a martial artist. After fifteen years of kick-boxing, ju-jitsu, and body building, the author decided to take her exploration of physical power to the next level, and she became a bouncer. Working the doors of club land provided her with the challenges she needed to put her martial arts skills to the test, as well as find out how, as a woman, she would react to both verbal, and physical, violence.

The seven years that were spent working as a bouncer were to prove illuminating. A fascination with the study of energy led to some of the roughest clubs in London, and beyond. It was by confronting violence, and not walking away from it, that the unexpected happened: an alternative to using force. Softness became the greatest ally, and opened the door to another world.

Softness was the greatest teacher, and it didn't take long to embody its power. Charly was, after all, no stranger to energetic healing: she had used vibrational medicine on family and friends as a child, and, throughout her life, has been called on to assist in the healing process of others.

Charly Flower now lives in England. She is a medicine woman, and has been practising as a soul doctor for many years. She offers sacred space to both women and men, and runs women-only workshops and drumming circles.

For any inquiries about this book, or for any information about Charly Flower's shamanic workshops and training for women, please email her at: charly.flower@yahoo.co.uk.
You can also visit her website: www.flowersoldier.com

Notes

Notes

Notes